DEVELOPMENT OF PSYCHO-MOTOR COMPETENCE

Selected Readings

Edited by
Linda Blane
University of Massachusetts

GENERAL EDITORS FOR THE SERIES

Daniel C. Jordan • Donald T. Streets

This is a custom-made book of readings prepared for the courses taught by the editors, as well as for related courses and for college and university libraries. For information about our program, please write to:

MSS INFORMATION CORPORATION
655 Madison Avenue
New York, New York 10021

MSS wishes to express its appreciation to the authors of the articles in this collection for their cooperation in making their work available in this format.

Library of Congress Cataloging in Publication Data

Blane, Linda, comp.
  Development of psycho-motor competence.

  CONTENTS: Introduction. — Balance and posture: Corballis, M. C. and Beale, I. L. Bilateral symmetry and behavior. Belmont, L. and Birch, H. G. Lateral dominance and right-left awareness in normal children. Cron, G. W. and Pronko, N. H. Development of the sense of balance in school children. Berman, A. Reliability of perceptual-motor laterality tasks. [etc.]
  1. Developmental psychobiology — Addresses, essays, lectures. 2. Psychomotor disorders — Addresses, essays, lectures. I. Jordan, Daniel C., joint comp. II. Streets, Donald T., joint comp. III. Title.
[DNLM: 1. Motor skills — Collected works. 2. Psychology, Educational — Colledted works.
WE103 B642d]
RJ131.B49   612'.76   74-31488
ISBN 0-8422-5219-3
ISBN 0-8422-0443-1 pbk.

CONTENTS

ACKNOWLEDGEMENTS

While developing the conceptual basis of the ANISA Model has been ten years in the making, the most productive period began in 1971 when the New England Program in Teacher Education, Durham, New Hampshire, granted nearly a quarter of a million dollars to the Center for the Study of Human Potential, School of Education, University of Massachusetts, for the purposes of completing the formulation of the theory which defines the Model and developing a teacher preparation program congruent with it. The grant provided the means for assembling a staff of graduate students and faculty most of whom have participated intensively for two to three years in developing the Model. While each volume in this series has been organized primarily by one or two people and the articles on Anisa have been written by one or more authors, all members of the staff have been involved in the development of the Model itself; thus, each volume represents a collective effort.

We are deeply grateful to the New England Program in Teacher Education and to the School of Education at the University of Massachusetts for their support and are eager to acknowledge the contributions of staff members and research associates of the ANISA Project staff, both past and present.

Among the most devoted and hardworking members of any enterprise like the Anisa project are the office personnel. Miss Sandra Rhode deserves special recognition for her willing and able administrative assistance to the project and Mrs. Edyth Overing for her careful preparation of manuscripts and the maintenance of bibliographies.

Mrs. Carla Jean Jeffords served as technical assistant and administrative coordinator for the publication of the series. We are especially tnankful for her impressive efficiency, her expertise in lay-out, printing, and publishing, and her helpful spirit.

Daniel C. Jordan
Donald T. Streets
General Editors for the Series

Amherst, Massachusetts
May 1974

PREFACE

What will the world we live in be like twenty-five years from now? What can we do now to prepare children for living then? The American Academy of Arts and Sciences' Commission on the Year 2000 sought answers to these questions. They analyzed current trends in social and technological development, attempted to identify the critical issues presently facing man, projected alternative futures, and suggested courses of action that would insure our survival as we approach the millenium. Throughout the report, the role of education was heavily implicated in any anticipated success as creating our own futures in ways that would not only guarantee our survival but also continually improve its quality. Yet, it was recognized that education itself must undergo radical changes if it is to play that role with any distinction.

> If we are to remain true to our democratic heritage one of the most obvious implications of the predictive increase in population is that our already crowded educational system will have to be vastly expanded and over-hauled...Put together the increased knowledge of students, the increased knowledge to be communicated, and the increased duration of the educational experience, and then try to imagine what kind of educational system we will need by the year 2000. Can anything short of an educational revolution meet our needs? (emphasis ours)

We believe that such expansion and overhauling are overdue and that nothing short of a revolution in education is required if we are to prepare children for the year 2000 and beyond. But revolutions can be haphazard, piece-meal, costly, inefficient and even destructive of elements of tradition which are essential to survival; or, they can be based on reason and science, carefully planned and executed, and therefore more constructive, more efficient and less costly.

The education professions' response to the crises in education has not been lacking, but to date it has been inadequate to initiate

---

[1]Miller, George A. "Some Psychological Perspectives on the Year 2000." DAEDALUS: Journal of the American Academy of Arts and Sciences, Summer 1967.

and sustain any revolution. Instead, it has been a mixture of highly theoretical and scientific efforts, on one hand, and a proliferation of programs and projects with little or no theoretical basis, on the other—the latter often reflecting an unjustifiable devotion to innovation for innovation's sake. Both the scientific efforts and the programs have been fragmented and piece-meal in nature, most of them hastily conceived, improperly researched, and costly.

To plan and carry forth a revolution of significance in education will depend on the identification of first principles of broad generality such that the massive amount of factual and theoretical information we have about human learning, growth, and development can be effectively integrated, programmatically applied, tested out, refined, and extended.

The development of the ANISA comprehensive educational Model* represents a decade-long effort to formulate such first principles and to derive a coherent body of theory concerning development, curriculum, pedagogy, administration and evaluation from these principles. Without theory there can be no science; without science there is little predictability; and without predictability there can be no accountability. Thus, we believe that this endeavor to formulate a comprehensive theory of education constitutes a significant step in the direction of establishing the bedrock on which education as a science may be built—a science which may guide and direct the needed expansion and overhauling of education and become the mainstay of a constructive and responsibly managed revolution.

This book of readings is one of many in a series designed to cover the main issues facing education as we move toward the year 2000 and beyond. The readings in each volume have been selected because they raise those critical issues and problems which any comprehensive theory of education must address. The final article in each book explains how the ANISA theory treats these issues and how it proposes to solve the problems they represent.

Taken as a whole, the series comprises enough material for a fairly comprehensive survey of the basic issues in the field of

*See Appendix for brief summary statement on the ANISA Model.

education; it also provides enough of a representative sampling of the many facets of the ANISA Model to reflect some of the promise we believe it holds for the systematic development of a science of education—ultimately the most compelling means of initiating and sustaining significant educational change.

Daniel C. Jordan, Director
Center for the Study
  of Human Potential

Donald T. Streets
Associate Director

INTRODUCTION

This volume is organized into six sections, each reflecting an area of concern within the domain of psycho-motor development. These sections are: (1) Balance and Posture; (2) Locomotion; (3) Manipulation; (4) Effecting Voluntary Control Over Visceral and Glandular Responses; (5) Plasticity of Psycho-Motor Competency; and, (6) A Proposal for a Comprehensive View of Psycho-Motor Development. Within the framework of this volume, psycho-motor competency is viewed as that ability to distinguish and bring under voluntary control (to the highest degree that is possible) those muscles and muscle groups which are mobilized to express the purposes of the organism in an infinitude of ways (combinations of movements).

Balance and Posture

Corbalis and Beale (1970) have formulated a promising hypothesis to account for the difficulty the human organism encounters in making lateral response differentiations (e.g., left from right). They build a compelling case for the position that man's physiological bilateral symmetry is responsible for mirror image reversals and that there is a transfer of learning (via the corpus callosum in the brain) from one side of the brain to the other to achieve functional symmetry.

Empirical evidence collected by Belmont and Birch (1963) indicate a developmental course (age specificity in lateral differentiations) in the discrimination of right-left relations (own body parts, body parts of others, object parts), eyedness and eye-hand preferences. They suggest that right-left discrimination of one's own body parts is independent of handedness. This study is suggestive of the existence of critical periods in the development of lateral differentiations.

Cron and Pronko (1957) make us acutely aware that although there may be developmental differences in balance (using a 12 foot board) among young (4 years) and older (15 years) children, other factors contribute to an individual child's psycho-motor performance. Some of these may be cultural differences in sex role expectations with respect to the task, competition, or presence or non-presence of an audience. These factors are of concern not only for the psycho-motor researcher but also for teachers who wish to arrange a specific environment and guide the learner's interactions with that environment for the purpose of developing his psycho-motor competence.

Assessment of "where the child is" is necessary for at lease three reasons: to effect an appropriate match between the learner's developmental level and the challenge of the learning experience; to assess the individual child's growth following a learning experience; and to establish age-related psycho-motor competence norms. Berman (1973) examines the test-retest reliability of several perceptual-motor laterality measures and discusses these findings with comments on research needs.

Locomotion

After observing seven children who were retarded in their developmental progress from locomotor immobility to skilled crawling, Freedman and Cannady (1971) confirmed the emergence of the crawling pattern as proposed by McGraw's (1941)* research. Freedman and Cannady's study lends support to the concept of a relatively fixed developmental sequence of steps in the development of prone locomotion. However, they suggest factors which may modify this sequence (cause a reversal in one or more stages in the sequence) and propose that the developmental process is not solely maturational.

Rhythmic accompaniment appears to facilitate the learning of specific motor skills of first through sixth graders (Beisman, 1967). This study provokes many questions: Are there correlations between the development of separate motor skills? Are there developmental trends in any such correlations? Are there sex differences in the development of skills using rhythm? Beisman directly or indirectly addresses some of these issues.

Manipulation

Manipulation of one's environment is only possible when one can first reach and successfully grasp the desired object, whether part of the external environment or one's own body. White, Castle and Held (1964) observed the emergence of visually directed prehension in infants during the first six

---

*McGraw, M. Development of neuro-muscular mechanisms as reflected in the crawling and creeping behavior of the human infant. J. Genet. Psychol., 1941, 58, 83-111.

months of life. They conclude that the process is sequential (eight stages, each approximately two weeks in duration) and propose that specific perceptual-motor matches (visual-motor and tactile-motor) are crucial in the development of prehension. They compel the reader to examine the importance of appropriate stimulation at the critical time. This, in turn, has strong implications for increasing the child's productive encounters with his environment as proposed later in this volume by Lietz (1972) and Dennis (1960).

Modeling, one of the most effective modes of teaching, rests on the learner's capacity to reproduce a movement exhibited by the teacher. Martiniuk, Shields, and Campbell (1972) explore those cues which are used in the reproduction of particular arm movements, manipulating a lever along an arc. They write:

". . . the starting and terminal positions of a movement were important cues in movement reproduction, whereas timing ability and movement velocity seemed unrelated to accuracy [p. 51].

Effecting Voluntary Control Over Visceral and Glandular Responses

There has long been evidence that conscious control can be exerted over large muscle groups. Basmajian (1963) demonstrated just how fine a motor discrimination and activation can be voluntarily made when auditory and visual cues (feedback) are present. Budzynski, Stoyva, and Adler (1970) further support the view that through the use of feedback conscious control over muscles and the subsequent reduction in headache can be facilitated.

The wealth of research concerning the voluntary control of muscles activating the skeletal system (see previous sections) has been accompanied by the assumption that visceral and glandular responses could not come under voluntary control. However, recent research (Miller, 1969; Shearn, 1961; Schwartz, 1972; Maslach, Marshall, and Zimbarlo, 1972) takes issue with this assertion. Miller's work demonstrates that the visceral and glandular systems can come under voluntary control in animals and, further, that the learning involved follows many of the same principles governing instrumental skeletal learning. Shearn indicates some tentative principles gleaned from the literature to account for changes in heart amplitude and rate when conditioned stimuli are present. He raises and discusses an interesting question: Does the heart learn? In a later study, Schwartz asserts that people can voluntarily control heart rate and systolic blood pressure (in tandem or separately) under conditions of feedback and reward. He proposes an explanatory model to account for this control. Here the reader has the opportunity to integrate the principles/ models proposed by these researchers. In their study, Maslach, Marshall, and Zimbarlo found that subjects who were trained under hypnosis were able to simultaneously obtain separate skin temperatures in their two hands. Wakeful subjects could not effect this difference. This study provokes the crucial question as to what types of learning experiences eventuate in voluntary control of the constriction of the walls of specific blood vessels.* Perhaps Miller's work has some bearing on this issue.

Plasticity of Psycho-Motor Development

While the reader will probably note that only two articles appear in this section of the readings, he should also be aware that there are implications for plasticity evident throughout the volume (Belmont and Birch, 1963; White, Castle and Held, 1964; Freedman and Cannady, 1971), in addition to the articles by Dennis (1960) and Lietz (1972). All these articles generate important questions concerning the issue of plasticity of psycho-motor development: Are there relatively fixed sequences in psycho-motor development? If the foregoing is the case, do sequences hold for all human beings, regardless of sex and race? Are there critical periods in the psycho-motor development where the absence of a critical learning experience results in a decrease in psycho-motor competency? What constitutes the best match between development and learning experience during a critical period if, indeed, they do exist? What does the foregoing imply concerning the time it takes an individual child to transverse a sequence? What are the implications of all of the above for the development of total learning competency?

A Proposal for a Comprehensive View of Psycho-Motor Competency

Blane and Jordan's (1974) article presents a developmental, theoretical model of psycho-motor competency as part of the comprehensive perspective of the ANISA Model. Developmental competency in the Model is presented in terms of the

---

*The dilation and constriction of the walls of the blood vessels controls the amount of blood flow in that particular area of the body which, in turn, determines the temperature of the surrounding body area.

processes which mediate the release of psycho-motor potentiality and is tied in with total human functioning. In his
article, Ausubel (1966) raises an important issue: Does
voluntary control of movement build, in part, upon reflexes
present at birth as Blane and Jordan's and Piaget's theories
propose? Ausubel suggests it does not.

Although this volume is organized according to the different processes which are evident in the growth of psycho-
motor competency, it should be remembered that the learner
himself remains an organized, functional unity. Thus, one is
continually impressed by the learner's integration of the
psycho-motor, volitional, perceptual, cognitive, and affective competencies to achieve maximal growth from any experience.

Linda M. Blane
Center for the Study of Human
    Potential
University of Massachusetts
Amherst, Massachusetts

PART I

BALANCE AND POSTURE

BILATERAL SYMMETRY AND BEHAVIOR[1]

M. C. CORBALLIS   AND   I. L. BEALE

Two tests of the ability to distinguish left from right, mirror-image stimulus discrimination and left-right response differentiation, are defined. A perfectly bilaterally symmetrical machine could perform neither test. Evidence is reviewed that animals and men find both tests difficult, especially the first. It is suggested that interhemispheric fiber systems (such as the corpus callosum) act to "symmetrize" memory traces and thus preserve structural symmetry. This may partly explain findings of mirror-image reversal accompanying interhemispheric transfer. Evidence is also described which suggests that animals may sometimes solve problems of mirror-image stimulus discrimination by adopting asymmetrical postures or by making asymmetrical responses in scanning the stimuli.

People often have difficulty telling which is left and which is right. Children, in particular, may have considerable difficulty establishing which is their left or right hand, and when they are learning to read or write, they often confuse letters, or even words, with their lateral mirror images. Many adults also confuse left and right. For example, Helmholtz was reputedly "left-right blind" to a considerable degree (Fritsch, 1968). There is also a growing literature which suggests that many animals have trouble with certain problems involving left and right.

The purpose of this article is to suggest that the problem of left and right is fundamentally related to the bilateral symmetry of the nervous system. This idea is one that can be traced to Ernst Mach (1894, 1959). He argued that a bilaterally symmetrical system, like the visual system in man, could not tell left from right, where each is defined relative to the system's plane of symmetry. The fact that man usually *can* distinguish left from right was merely evidence that asymmetry existed somewhere in the nervous system. Mach (1959) thought that this asymmetry was motor

rather than sensory. He wrote:

After the space sensations of the eye have become associated, through writing, with the right hand, a confusion of those vertically symmetrical figures with which the art and habit of writing are concerned no longer ensues [p. 111].

But, he added,

The confusion of right and left [still] occurs . . . with regard to figures which have no motor, but only a purely optical (for example, ornamental) interest [p. 111].

Mach's views have been largely overlooked by recent authors writing on the problem, though there are exceptions (e.g., Noble, 1966, 1968; Tschirgi, 1958). However, there are logical as well as empirical grounds for supposing that left-right confusion is indeed a consequence of bilateral symmetry. There is also some recent support for Mach's contention that response asymmetries may play a crucial role in the discrimination of mirror-image stimuli. The present authors' purpose is to develop these ideas in some detail. Many of the conclusions will be speculative, and some of them conflict with alternative ideas as to why left-right confusions are so common. Therefore, we hope that this article will at least serve to encourage further research on this ubiquitous problem.

TELLING LEFT FROM RIGHT

There are two ways to decide whether an animal can tell left from right. One is to

[1] This work was partially supported by grants from the American Psychological Foundation and from the National Research Council of Canada to the first author. The authors are indebted to many people, most especially to D. Bindra, D. O. Hebb, R. J. Irwin, R. Melzack, P. M. Milner, J. Noble, R. Over, and N. S. Sutherland, for helpful comments.

determine if the animal can *decode* a left-right difference in the environment by making responses that are *not* bilateral mirror images of one another to stimuli that *are* bilateral mirror images of one another. This is a test of *mirror-image discrimination.* Examples are (*a*) a man who says "left" or "right" when touched on the left or right side, (*b*) a pigeon which pecks a key when it displays a 135° line but does not peck when it displays a 45° line, or (*c*) a dog which salivates when touched on the left flank but does not salivate when touched on the homologous point on the right flank.

The second way is to enquire if the animal can *encode* a stimulus which contains no explicit left-right information by making either a left or a right response. This shall be called *left-right response differentiation.* The simplest kind is that in which no stimulus discrimination is required, as when a rat always turns left, say, in a symmetrical T maze. A more compelling test, however, is one in which the animal must make a left response to one stimulus and a right response to another, where the stimuli differ only in respects other than laterality. Examples include (*a*) a person who is instructed "turn left" or "turn right" and responds accordingly, (*b*) a dog which lifts its left paw when a buzzer sounds and its right paw when a bell rings, or (*c*) a monkey which chooses a left food box when a light is on and a right food box when the light is off.

It is important to note that a test in which an animal makes mirror-image responses to mirror-image stimuli cannot be construed as evidence that the animal can tell left from right in either of the above senses. Such a test requires neither decoding nor encoding of left-right information. Rather, the left-right information is simply transmitted, or copied, from stimuli to responses. The following examples, therefore, do *not* prove the ability to distinguish left from right: (*a*) a cat which scratches its left or right ear when it itches, (*b*) a rat which always turns into the lighted arm of a T maze, or (*c*) a man steering a car to the left or right to follow the curves in the road. In these examples, the responses have "told"

nothing of the difference between left and right beyond that which was already represented in the stimuli.

Restrictions Imposed by Bilateral Symmetry

Consider a bilaterally symmetrical machine which is constructed to respond to certain stimuli. A bilaterally symmetrical machine is one which is unchanged by mirror reflection. Examples which at least approximate symmetry are a wheelbarrow, a rolling pin, an aeroplane. Such a machine *must* make mirror-image responses to stimuli which are mirror images about its plane of symmetry. One way to see that this is so is to note that mirror reflection leaves the machine unaltered but converts any given stimulus and its response to their mirror images. Thus, the mirror representation shows that the same machine would make the mirror-image response to the mirror-image stimulus.[3] This means that a bilaterally symmetrical machine could not tell left from right. It could not discriminate mirror-image stimuli because it could not respond to them by giving differential responses which were *not* mirror images of one another. Neither could it differentiate left from right responses, because it must make symmetrical responses to symmetrical stimuli, which means that it could not make left or right responses in the absence of left-right information.

Assuming that an organism can be regarded as no more than a complex machine, these arguments must apply equally to a bilaterally symmetrical organism as to a bilaterally symmetrical machine. On purely mechanical grounds, then, it can be asserted that a perfectly bilaterally symmetrical organism could not tell left from right. Now, no real organism is *perfectly* bilaterally symmetrical—a matter we shall take up later— but most organisms are approximately so. This, we propose, is why they often find it at least difficult to tell left from right.

[3] Strictly, this is so only if parity is conserved; that is, if the laws of nature remain unaltered by mirror reflection. We therefore ignore the possible consequences of the discovery by physicists that parity is in certain instances not conserved.

It is also true that one can seldom, if ever, find stimuli which are *exact* mirror images with respect to animal's midsagittal plane (which can be taken, at least approximately, to be its plane of symmetry). However, in tests of mirror-image discrimination, we need only require that the animal be able to discriminate between two sets of stimuli which are mirror images *on the average,* such that the mirror image of any member of one set is at least potentially a member of the other. If the animal can reliably discriminate between such sets, then we can be reasonably sure it is in fact capable of exact mirror-image discrimination (and is, therefore, in some respect, asymmetrical). However, one must be careful to avoid constant asymmetrical features in the environment which might serve as left-right cues, such as a window in one wall, or noise from apparatus placed to one side, or the experimenter himself who may constantly observe from one side.

Similarly, in testing left-right response differentiation, we need not insist that individual stimuli be perfectly symmetrical, or carry absolutely no left-right information. However, there must be no *systematic* bias. If the command "left turn" always came from the left, and "right turn" always from the right, a symmetrical soldier would have no difficulty. But if each command is as likely to come from one side as from the other, a symmetrical soldier would not know which way to turn. It is said that soldiers in Czarist Russia solved this problem by wearing a bundle of hay tied to the left leg and a bundle of straw tied to the right, and were thus provided with a constant asymmetrical cue (Fritsch, 1968, p. 55).

EXPERIMENTAL EVIDENCE

Mirror-Image Discrimination

Many species find it at least difficult, sometimes impossible, to discriminate between mirror-image stimuli. For example, Pavlov (1927) wrote that it was virtually impossible to condition a dog to salivate when touched on one side of the body but not to salivate when touched on the homologous point on the other side. Tschirgi (1958) states that a cat cannot be taught to choose a circle when touched on one side of the body and a square when touched on the other side. Other tests show that the cat can discriminate a circle from a square, so the problem seems to be that it cannot distinguish the mirror-image touches. However, cats can readily learn to discriminate between rectangles oriented at 45° and 135° to the horizontal (Sutherland, 1963). Children (Rudel & Teuber, 1963) and octopuses (Sutherland, 1960), though, apparently find it practically impossible to discriminate between mirror-image obliques. Rats (Lashley, 1938), goldfish (Mackintosh & Sutherland, 1963), monkeys (Riopelle, Itoigawa, Rahm, & Draper, 1964), and chimpanzees (Nissen & McCulloch, 1937) also have trouble discriminating between certain pairs of lateral mirror images.

We can draw a distinction between successive discrimination, in which the stimuli are presented one at a time, and simultaneous discrimination, in which both are presented at once and the animal must choose between them. Simultaneous discrimination of mirror-image pairs requires further comment, because if the stimuli are arranged side by side, the test can be interpreted as one of left-right response differentiation rather than mirror-image stimulus discrimination. Stimuli that are lateral mirror images of one another form a bilaterally symmetrical pair if they are placed side by side, so that an animal that learns to choose between them could be learning to go left to one symmetrical combination, right to the other. For example, suppose an animal is confronted simultaneously with a 45° line and a 135° line and is required to select the 135° line. It might learn to respond correctly by selecting the right-hand line when the two lines converge upward, and the left-hand line when they converge downward. However, there is evidence that both cats (Sutherland, 1963) and pigeons (Corballis & Beale, 1967), after learning to discriminate mirror-image obliques presented simultaneously, continue to choose correctly when the stimuli are presented one at a time. This suggests that simultaneous discrimination of mirror-image pairs involves genuine mirror-image discrimination, rather than left-right response differentiation. That is, in simultaneous discrimination, animals probably do not respond on the basis of the entire stimulus complex, but attend rather to the individual stimuli one at a time.

Left-Right Response Differentiation

Tests of left-right response differentiation per se seem to be few. Konorski (1964), though not explicitly concerned with this problem, reported that dogs were unable to learn to go to a left food tray in response to one sound and to a right food tray in response to another. In another experiment, it proved impossible to teach a dog to lift its right foreleg in response to a metronome and its left foreleg in response to a buzzer. In both cases, however, failure to learn the differentiation only occurred when the stimuli sounded from the same position. When the sounds came from sources in different spatial positions the animal readily learned the differentiation. Konorski does not give details of the symmetry of the positioning of the sound sources, but we may surmise that when they were in different positions, the spatial origin of each provided the left-right cue. It should be noted that dogs were easily able to discriminate the sounds used in these experiments when tested in classical conditioning or "go–no go" paradigms. The problem in the "go left–go right" paradigm therefore seems to be one of response differentiation, not of stimulus discrimination.

As was noted earlier, the simplest kind of left-right response differentiation is that in which no stimulus discrimination is involved at all. This does not appear to be a particularly difficult task. For example, Grindley (1932) found that guinea pigs could be taught to turn their heads to one side in response to a buzzer. Moreover, rats can learn to choose one arm of a T maze for food reward in the absence of any stimulus cues as to which is the correct arm. However, they cannot learn more complex mazes involving left-right choices unless there are external left-right cues, and they learn simple mazes more easily if such cues are present (Restle, 1957).

There is at least anecdotal evidence that young children find it difficult to differentiate right from left. Hebb (1949) writes of

the notorious difficulty of choosing between *left* and *right*, to be observed by anyone who tries to teach twelve-year old children to "right turn" promptly on command [p. 118].

The problem is clearly not one of discriminating the stimuli, for, as Hebb puts it, "The child can readily learn at the age of three that 'right' and 'left' each refers to a side of the body—but ah me, which one [p. 118]?" Young children also often write letters, or even words, backwards. It is of interest that reading and writing difficulties are much rarer among Japanese children than among Western children. This as been partly attributed to the fact that any symbol in Japanese script can be written in mirror-image form and still be recognized as having the same meaning, whereas b and d, p and q, MAY and YAM, etc., have very different meanings in English script (Makita, 1968).

Symmetry, Learning, and the Corpus Callosum

The examples cited show that animals do not merely have difficulty distinguishing between left and right, they also have difficulty *learning* to do so. This suggests that they tend to remain structurally symmetrical, more or less, in spite of asymmetrical training. The corpus callosum may be crucial in preserving symmetry during learning. Evidence for this comes from an early split-brain experiment described by Pavlov. It had been found practically impossible to condition a dog to salivate when touched on one side of the body but not when touched on the mirror-image locus on the other side. To explore this phenomenon further, one of Pavlov's co-workers, Bikov, sectioned the corpus callosum. When this was done, conditioned responses to touches on either side of the body became entirely independent, so that the mirror-image discrimination was easily established (Pavlov, 1927, p. 352).

These findings can be readily understood in terms of homotopic interhemispheric connections. There is evidence, from subhuman species at least, that each cerebral hemisphere is the mirror image of the other, and that callosal and commissural fibers between the hemispheres connect mirror-image points (e.g., Grafstein, 1959; Morrell, 1963; Sperry, 1962). Thus, an animal learning to respond to a touch on the right side also learns to respond identically to a touch on the left side, because the central locus corresponding to a right-side touch is connected interhemispherically to the equivalent central locus corresponding to a left-side touch. This argument is readily extended to any pair of stimuli which are mirror images with respect to the animal's midsagittal plane. Hence, the action of the corpus callosum, and possibly of other interhemispheric fibers as well, may be to "symmetrize" memory traces, to preserve the symmetry of structural changes which may occur in learning, and thus make it difficult or impossible for the animal to learn a mirror-image discrimination.

Of course, not all cortical activity is symmetrized. For example, callosal connections in the visual cortex of cat (Choudhury, Whitteridge, & Wilson, 1965) and monkey (Myers, 1962) seem to be lacking in area 19 and most of area 17. Moreover, in the cat, at least, there appear to be fibers from the lateral part of area 17 on one side which connect to area 18 on the other side (Hubel & Wiesel, 1967), and these connections are clearly *not* between mirror-image points. However, callosal connections in the visual cortex are probably not concerned with transfer of learning, but rather with preserving the continuity of the visual field across the vertical meridian (Hubel & Wiesel, 1967; Whitteridge, 1965).

It may be helpful at this point to draw a distinction between, on the one hand, perceptual and short-term memory processes which depend on only temporary neural activity, and on the other hand, long-term memory processes which result in more or less permanent structural changes (e.g., Hebb, 1949). There seems good reason to believe that the latter may be symmetrized, but that the former need not be. Indeed it would be a severe disadvantage if perceptual processes *were* symmetrized, for this would deprive the animal of any asymmetrical in-

formation at all. It would never know, for example, which car to scratch if one of them itched, or which way to turn if threatened from one side or the other. All animals have the ability to respond asymmetrically in the presence of asymmetrical information, so they must possess the mechanisms to at least perceive such information.

Two studies using mirror-image stimuli with children illustrate this difference between learning and perceptual processes. In one study, Jeffrey (1958) reported that children could not learn to give different verbal responses to each of a lateral mirror-image pair of pointing stick figures. However, they could readily learn to press buttons oriented in the directions indicated by the pointing figures, which means they could at least *perceive* the asymmetry in the figures and match it with that of the response buttons. In a similar study, Over and Over (1967) found that young children could not learn to recognize and consistently select one of two mirror-image oblique lines, but they could easily tell whether two oblique lines were the same or whether they were mirror images of one another. Recognition requires that the child learn and *remember* an association to one of the lines but not to its mirror image. This may have been impossible because of the symmetrization of the memory trace. However, judgments of sameness or difference depend simply on the matching of percepts or short-term memory traces, which need not imply structural change. We suggest, then, that children may perceive asymmetry, but may have great difficulty remembering an asymmetrical stimulus as being distinct from its lateral mirror image.

The interhemispheric transfer of learning may not always be total. In the pigeon, both color and pattern discrimination learning transfer more or less completely from one hemisphere to the other (Mello, 1968). In cats (Myers, 1957) and monkeys (Downer, 1962), however, it appears that transfer is less complete, especially for relatively difficult discriminations. The extent to which structural traces are symmetrized may therefore depend on the difficulty of the discrimination and perhaps also on the level of complexity of the organism. We shall argue later that symmetrization may be important mainly to creatures which are relatively stimulus bound, whose nervous systems are mainly concerned with movement and orientation in a more or less symmetrical world. But for higher organisms, capable of manipulative behavior and symbolic thought, we shall suggest that symmetrization may be a disadvantage.

Interhemispheric Mirror-Image Reversal

If the two hemispheres are mirror images of one another, and if interhemispheric fibers do indeed connect mirror-image points, then a rather surprising consequence follows. Interhemispheric transfer, when it does occur, should be accompanied by mirror-image reversal. That is, if one hemisphere records a habit to turn left, the other should register a habit to turn right; if a 45° line is of significance to one hemisphere, a 135° line should be of equal significance to the other. Most investigators have studied the interhemispheric transfer of symmetrical habits, so the possibility of reversal does not arise. However, there are experiments on the interhemispheric transfer of both mirror-image discrimination and left-right response differentiation which suggest that reversal does indeed occur, although the explanation for this is not always unequivocal.

Ray and Emley (1964, 1965) have examined the interhemispheric transfer of a left-right response differentiation in rats. The animals were trained to turn into one arm of a T maze when a light was on, and into the other arm when the light was off. During training, one cortical hemisphere was functionally depressed by the application of KCl solution. After training, the rats were given one test trial with the other hemisphere depressed. Half of the animals were tested with the light on and half with it off. Nearly all responded by running into the arm of the T maze that was *opposite* to the one they had learned during training. Correct differentiation was restored on the following trial when the original hemisphere was again depressed. Mirror-image reversal also occurred on a later transfer trial which followed a trial with both hemispheres functional, but only when the interval between these trials was short (15 seconds). If the application of KCl for the transfer trial was delayed 10 or 30 minutes after the trial with both hemispheres functional, there was no reversal.

One curious feature of these results is that mirror-image reversal occurred on the very first transfer trial. It is not obvious how transfer occurred at all, let alone reversal of it, since the hemisphere that was tested had always been depressed during learning. It is possible that depression was not total, and that transfer did occur cortically, but that the depression was sufficient to block the (mirror-image) *response* from the depressed hemisphere. This suggests, incidentally, that an animal with one hemisphere depressed ought to be able to learn a left-right differentiation more easily than one with both hemispheres intact, since such an animal is effectively, though temporarily, asymmetrical. In effect, left-right differentiation may be possible *because* the mirror-image response is blocked.

There is some evidence for interhemispheric reversal of mirror-image discrimination in monkeys. Ettlinger and Elithorn (1962) trained monkeys to discriminate tactually the letter "C" from its mirror image, using one hand only. With the other hand, it then proved easier for the monkeys to learn the reverse discrimination than the original one. Initial responding with the untrained hand was at chance level, however. Noble (1966, 1968) has obtained similar results in the visual modality, using monkeys with split optic chiasms. The monkeys were trained monocularly to discriminate a number of pairs of lateral mirror images. When tested with the untrained eye, they displayed a preference for the previously negative stimulus. Again, however, this preference did not appear on initial transfer trials, but developed with subsequent testing. Noble recognized that this mirror-image reversal could be explained in terms of homotopic connections between hemispheres.

There is also some evidence for interocular mirror-image reversal in both goldfish (Ingle, 1967) and pigeons (Mello,

23

1965, 1966a, 1966b). It does not always occur in either species; in goldfish, Ingle found that the stimuli must exceed a certain size for reversal to occur, and Mello (1966a) found with pigeons that for certain mirror-image pairs there was lack of transfer rather than reversal. In both goldfish and pigeons, each eye projects wholly to the opposite hemisphere, so that interocular transfer is equivalent to interhemispheric transfer. Thus interocular mirror-image reversal in either species might be interpreted to mean that interhemispheric transfer is accompanied by mirror-image reversal of the memory trace.

However, there is a simpler explanation for Mello's results, an explanation which may or may not apply to species other than the pigeon. Mello used the standard operant apparatus for pigeons, in which a pigeon must peck a small circular key to obtain access to food. Pigeons trained monocularly to peck the key when it displayed one stimulus tended to peck more often at the lateral mirror image of that stimulus when tested with the untrained eye open. Now, a monocular pigeon tends to peck to one side of the key, the side of the seeing eye (Beale & Corballis, 1967, 1968).[4] This probably means that a bird viewing with its left eye responds on the basis of cues on the left of the key only, while a bird viewing with its right eye responds only to cues on the right. For example, suppose a bird viewing with its right eye only is taught to peck when a 135° line (S+) is displayed on the key, but not to peck when a 45° line (S−) is displayed. If the bird responds on the basis of cues on the right of the key only, then the discrimination might be effectively an up-down one rather than a mirror-image one, because on the right half of the key,

[4] Laterally displaced pecking in monocular pigeons bears some resemblance to the circling behavior exhibited by monocular insects, rabbits, and kittens, which is also toward the seeing eye (Walk, 1968). It may also be related to the fact that monocular pigeons fail to show an optokinetic reflex to stimuli moving from the nasal to the temporal field of the open eye (Huizinga & Van der Meulen, 1951). This could mean that they are partially deprived of visual feedback while pecking, producing "overshoot" toward the open eye.

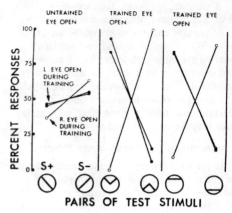

FIG. 1. Three birds were trained monocularly on a variable-interval schedule to peck to a 135° line (S+) but not to a 45° line (S−). (Figure shows percentage of responses on nonreinforced test discriminations. All birds were trained to a criterion of 90% correct responses before and between test trials. The eye that was open during training and testing, and the stimuli used in the test trials, are indicated. The data suggest that the birds discriminated the stimuli on the basis of up-down cues.)

the 135° line occupies the lower quadrant and the 45° line, the upper quadrant. Data summarized in Figure 1 show that birds taught monocularly to discriminate mirror-image obliques do in fact respond on the basis of up-down cues (Corballis & Beale, 1970).

If the bird that was trained with its right eye open is now tested with its left eye open, it should peck on the left of the key. Here, the line that occupies the lower quadrant is S−, the 45° line. Therefore, we might expect the bird to peck more often to S− than to S+, displaying mirror-image reversal. Similar explanations can be advanced for other mirror-image pairs. Thus interocular mirror-image reversal can be explained by supposing that pigeons peck on opposite sides of the key, depending on which eye is open; in other words, reversal depends on "beak shift" (Beale & Corballis, 1968).

We emphasize at this point that interocular mirror-image reversal, whatever the explanation for it, is exactly what one would expect of a bird that is bilaterally symmetrical. It can be interpreted as *failure* to dis-

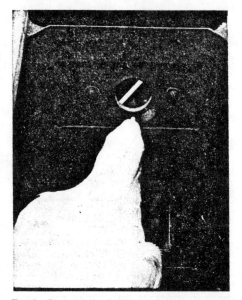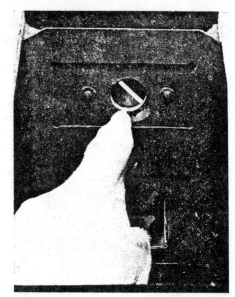

FIG. 2. Photograph of a pigeon tilting its head while pecking at 135° (S+) and 45° (S−) lines. (The effect of the head tilt is to transform the discrimination to a horizontal-vertical one.)

criminate between mirror-image stimuli. This is so because the lateral mirror image of a given pattern viewed through one eye is the left-right reflection of that pattern *viewed through the other eye,* if the plane of reflection is taken to be the bird's midsagittal plane. Mello's pigeons were effectively treating these mirror-image stimuli as though they were the same. Therefore, any bird which did *not* show interocular mirror-image reversal, but pecked instead to the same stimulus regardless of which eye was open, could be said to exhibit genuine mirror-image discrimination. Such a bird would be behaving asymmetrically.

Now, in both Mello's experiments and our own there were usually some birds which showed veridical interocular transfer rather than mirror-image reversal. We found that such birds tended not to display beak shift (Beale & Corballis, 1968). During testing with the untrained eye open, they generally continued to peck on the *same* side of the key that they had favored during training. This enabled them to correctly discriminate mirror-image obliques, probably in terms of up-down cues, regardless of which eye was

open. In other words, they had apparently acquired a response asymmetry which enabled them to perform a genuine mirror-image discrimination.

Role of Response Asymmetry in Mirror-Image Discrimination

Response asymmetry may play a rather general role in mirror-image discrimination, as Mach (1894, 1959) long ago conjectured. We have observed that pigeons taught to discriminate mirror images with *both* eyes open develop marked postural asymmetries. For example, one pigeon which we filmed extensively learned to discriminate mirror-image obliques by tilting its head to the right, so that the positive stimulus, a 135° line, became horizontal with respect to the bird's head, while the 45° line became vertical. This is shown in Figure 2. By adopting this asymmetrical posture, the pigeon was able to translate axes so that the mirror-image problem was converted, in the bird's eye view, into a horizontal-vertical one.

In another experiment, two pigeons were trained with both eyes open to peck a key

25

when the right half was blue and the left half red, but not to peck when the left half was blue and the right half red. The birds learned this discrimination by standing to one side and pecking on the half of the key to that side only. One bird stood to the left, the other to the right. Figure 3 shows generalization gradients obtained with both halves of the key the same color. It is clear that the first bird gave most responses when the key was red and fewest when it was blue, while the second pecked most to the blue and least to the red. Thus, by positioning themselves asymmetrically with respect to the key and ignoring one half of it, both birds were able to transform the discrimination from a mirror-image one to a simple color discrimination (Clarke, 1969).

Clearly, more research is needed to determine whether asymmetrical responses play a role in mirror-image discrimination in species other than the pigeon, and if so, what form they take. One might expect interspecies differences. For example, head tilt might explain why pigeons can so readily discriminate mirror-image obliques, but we doubt that it would be of much assistance to the octopus. The slitlike eye of the octopus is maintained in a horizontal position regardless of the orientation of its head or body (Young, 1962), so that head tilt would not cause rotation of the stimuli relative to the animal's eye. This might explain why octopuses find it much more difficult to discriminate mirror-image obliques than do cats, for example (cf. Sutherland, 1963).

The role of response asymmetry in mirror-image discrimination would surely depend on sense modality For visually presented stimuli, for example, the animal is usually free to move relative to the stimulus source, and so translate the stimuli relative to its own axes. But for tactile stimuli, say, this is generally not possible. One can touch an animal at mirror-image points relative to its midsagittal plane more or less regardless of the posture adopted by the animal. This could explain why both cats (Tschirgi, 1958) and dogs (Pavlov, 1927) apparently find it extremely difficult to discriminate a touch on one side of the body from a touch on the other side, while cats, at least, can

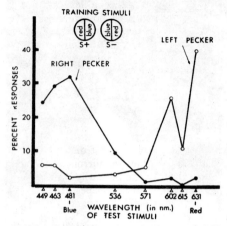

FIG. 3. Two birds were trained on a variable-interval schedule, with both eyes open, to peck when the key was red on the left and blue on the right, but not when it was blue on the left and red on the right. (Generalization gradients obtained under test conditions with no reinforcement, and with the key all one color, show that the discrimination was based on the colors appearing on one half of the key only.)

easily discriminate mirror-image obliques presented visually (Sutherland, 1963).

In man, left-to-right eye movements constitute an obvious means of discriminating between visual patterns that are mirror images of one another. If scanned from left to right b's and d's are no longer mirror images in spatiotemporal coordinates. Left-to-right scanning does not necessarily imply overt eye movements, as studies of tachistoscopic perception show (Bryden, 1961), but it probably originated in overt eye movements. With extensive practice, in reading, for example, the processes of visual attention may become "semiautonomous," or partially independent of eye movements (Hebb, 1963). Handedness probably also plays a role in the development of mirror-image discrimination, since we tend to manipulate the environment with one hand, usually the right, in preference to the other.

We are suggesting, then, that animals and men might sometimes solve problems of mirror-image discrimination by making asymmetrical responses. Such responses represent the simplest kind of left-right response differentiation, in which the animal always chooses either a left- or a right-oriented response or posture regardless of which stimulus is present. In short, all that is required is a constant, left or right response bias. Hand preference in humans is a good example, for it applies in practically all situations requiring the use of only one hand.

Alternative Theories

There are some alternative theories as to why some animals find it difficult or impossible to discriminate mirror-image stimuli. These theories are primarily concerned with the analysis of visual shapes. For example, Sutherland (1957) has suggested that the octopus analyzes shapes primarily in terms of their horizontal projections. Hence, it cannot discriminate mirror images because mirror-image shapes have identical horizontal projections. Dodwell (1957) proposed that rats analyze shapes in terms of the directions of their contours with respect to horizontal and vertical, and since 45° and 135° lines, for example, are both midway between horizontal and vertical, they would be indistinguishable. A closely related idea is that the ability to distinguish lines or rectangles in different orientations depends on the relative number of cells in the visual cortex sensitive to each orientation (Sutherland, 1963). This could explain why cats find it easy and octopuses difficult to discriminate mirror-image obliques, since cats appear to have as many cells sensitive to oblique lines as to horizontal and vertical lines (Hubel & Wiesel, 1962), while the visual system of the octopus seems primarily organized to detect horizontal and vertical only (Young, 1962). Finally, Deutsch (1955) has outlined a theory in which spatial patterns are transformed by the brain into temporal patterns, and it is a consequence of this theory that mirror-image shapes will give rise to identical temporal patterns.

These theories, we think, fail to capture the very general nature of the problem of distinguishing between left and right. They do not necessarily contradict, but neither do they consider the possibility that the difficulty with mirror-image discrimination is fundamentally related to bilateral symmetry. Our chief objection, however, is that all of them stress the loss of left-right information in *perceptual* analysis, whereas we have argued that left-right information is lost in the symmetrization of *memory* traces. For reasons already stated, we think it extremely unlikely, in general, that animals cannot perceive asymmetry, although it is conceivably true for certain visual shapes.

Over (1967) has made the valuable point that mirror-image discrimination experiments of the kind we have been considering do not allow a distinction between perceptual and memory processes, and therefore do not provide unequivocal information about the analysis of shapes as distinct from memory of them. Tests of oddity discrimination, matching to sample, or same-different judgments, using mirror-image stimuli, would provide more critical evidence of the ability of animals simply to detect left-right information. We have already described the experiments by Jeffrey (1958) and Over and Over (1967) suggesting that children can perform such tasks, but cannot accomplish mirror-image discriminations which require that they remember which stimulus is which. We suspect the same would often be true of animals. We also suspect that animals would have relatively little difficulty learning to make mirror-image respones to mirror-image stimuli, since this would also require perception but not memory of left-right information; it does not constitute genuine mirror-image discrimination. The theories described above, by contrast, imply that all of these tasks would be difficult or impossible.

On the Symmetry of Organisms

The main thesis of this article is that a bilaterally symmetrical organism cannot tell left from right. This is of practical importance only to the extent that real organisms are bilaterally symmetrical. In this section, we comment more specifically on bilateral symmetry, and departures from it, in the structure of biological systems.

First, bilateral symmetry is not a necessary quality of living organisms. Indeed, Louis Pasteur was long ago struck by the fact that the *molecules* of living tissue are asymmetrical, and even considered asymmetry a possible defining characteristic of living as opposed to inorganic matter (e.g., Gardner, 1964, Ch. 12). The DNA molecule, for example, like the corkscrew, is a right-handed helix. Here we may remark that mirror-image discrimination is readily achieved at the molecular level, as we might expect from the structural asymmetry of organisms at this level. Chemical stereoisomers, whose molecules are mirror images of one another, often taste and smell different from one another. For example, geraniol smells like roses while its stereoisomer smells like fresh oil. Also, levorotatory camphor is lethal to dogs and rabbits, but dextrorotatory camphor is relatively harmless (Fritsch, 1968, p. 119).

Bilateral symmetry, then, appears at higher levels than the molecular, although even here there are striking exceptions, such as right- and left-handed helical shells, the fiddler crab with one large and one small pincer, and the anableps—the remarkable four-eyed fish with sex organs on one side of the body. (These, and other examples are given in Gardner, 1964.) In man there are several departures from bilateral symmetry in the placement of the internal organs. The heart and stomach are displaced to the left, the liver and appendix to the right, an arrangement that presumably makes for more efficient packaging than symmetrical placement. But still, the overriding impression in most species, including man, is one of structural symmetry rather than asymmetry, especially with regard to external appearances, the placement of sensory organs and motor apparatus, and the structure of the central nervous system.

Broadly speaking, the evolutionary development of the nervous system can be seen as a progression from spherical symmetry, to radial symmetry, to bilateral symmetry, and perhaps to the emergence of asymmetry in man (Tschirgi, 1958). Symmetry probably has survival value at different levels. The spherically symmetrical organisms were small creatures suspended in the ocean depths, where environmental forces were as likely to act in one direction as another.

Consequently, it would have been of advantage to such a creature to be equally sensitive in all directions. In shallower waters or on land, gravity provides a uniform directional influence giving rise to an up-down axis, but radial symmetry could still be important. However, radial symmetry probably gave way to bilateral symmetry as organisms evolved the capacity to move, since linear movement is most efficiently accomplished by a system that is bilaterally symmetrical (Weyl, 1953). Even though motor systems in some cases evolved independently of one another, legs, fins, flippers, and wings are nearly always organized symmetrically (Gardner, 1964, Ch. 7). (Curiously enough, however, the gallop of a horse is asymmetrical.)

Linear movement and the development of bilaterally symmetrical motor systems probably presaged the bilaterally symmetrical placement of sense organs. Sensory information is involved in movement in many obvious ways, in feedback, for example. Further, for an organism moving in a straight line, environmental influences from front and back would no longer be equal, but there would still be no overall bias from one or the other *side*. Reward or threat are equally likely to appear from left or right. Hence the sense organs are best placed symmetrically with respect to the midline. Symmetry of sensory and motor systems probably dictated the symmetry of at least the greater part of the central nervous system. These points are more fully discussed by Gardner (1964, Ch. 7).

But another development occurred as the precursors of man evolved an upright stance. The hands were no longer required for locomotion and could be used for manipulating the environment. Here, bilateral symmetry may have been a disadvantage, since many manipulations, especially those involving the use of tools, require that one hand hold while the other operate. Examples are hammering, chopping, cutting, stirring, writing, and changing diapers on a small but active child. Hence, in man, one hand assumed "dominance" over the other. It has been suggested that man became right-handed because he held his shield in his left hand in order to protect his heart, which is slightly to the left of midline, so that it was the right hand which wielded the sword (Stier, 1911, cited by Von Bonin, 1962).

Bruner (1969) has pointed out that the relation between holding and operating is analogous to that between topic and comment in language. This relation is essentially that of predication. Asymmetry in intermanual functions may therefore have set the stage for the cortical asymmetry of function that is characteristic of language representation in the human brain. The nondominant hemisphere, Bruner suggests, may be more or less responsible for holding or preserving context, while the dominant hemisphere produces the focal operations, the actual speech.

Gazzaniga (1968) has also speculated about the relation between handedness and cerebral dominance. He cites evidence that the corpus callosum in man develops relatively late, so that young children are effectively "split-brained." This means that in right-handed children structural traces will be elaborated more in the left hemisphere than in the right. Symmetrization cannot occur because the corpus callosum is lacking. Elaboration of the left hemisphere leads to increased use of the right hand, so the effect is cumulative. Therefore, the left hemisphere may be developed to the extent that it can accommodate the complexity of speech mechanisms, whereas the right hemisphere is not.

Whatever the force of these speculations by Bruner and by Gazzaniga, there is reason to believe that symbolic thought processes, like certain bimanual skills, might be hindered by symmetrization. For one thing, it seems a sheer waste of storage space to have memories duplicated (mirror-wise) in each hemisphere, and storage capacity probably became increasingly important as the brain evolved more symbolic and less stimulus-bound functions. Second, it could be a disadvantage not to be able to tell left from right. Many of the symbolic behaviors developed by man, from shaking hands to reading and writing, exploit the left-right dimension in a way that would be impossible if man's brain were bilaterally symmetrical.

There is increasing documentation of lateralization of function in the brain of man, much of it related to language representation (e.g., Gazzaniga & Sperry, 1967; Millikan & Darley, 1967; Mountcastle, 1962). And as one might expect, there is relatively little evidence for cerebral asymmetry in other species (though perhaps this is because researchers have not really looked for it). However, Trevarthen (1970) has found evidence for spontaneous lateralization of the processes regulating a complex, learned manipulative skill in the baboon. The skill was a bilaterally symmetrical one requiring fine finger movements of both hands. Thus, the mechanisms for cerebral lateralization of function might already be partially formed in subhuman primates.

Much of this discussion of symmetry and asymmetry in evolution has been frankly speculative, and has overlooked important issues. Moreover, the dangers of inferring evolutionary changes by comparing living animals have been well stated by Hodos and Campbell (1969). Our main point, however, is simply that the symmetries that are so prevalent in living organisms probably result mainly from lack of directional biases in the physical environment. But with the evolution of functions that are not tied to the immediate environment, there need no longer be any pressure toward symmetry; in fact, symmetry may often be a disadvantage. However, even man is more obviously symmetrical than he is asymmetrical, and even man occasionally confuses left and right.

REFERENCES

BEALE, I. L., & CORBALLIS, M. C. Laterally displaced pecking in monocularly viewing pigeons: A possible factor in interocular mirror-image reversal. *Psychonomic Science*, 1967, 9, 603–604.

BEALE, I. L., & CORBALLIS, M. C. Beak shift: An explanation for interocular mirror-image reversal in pigeons. *Nature*, 1968, 220, 82–83.

BRUNER, J. Up from helplessness. *Psychology Today*, 1969, 2(June), 30.

BRYDEN, M. P. The role of post-exposural eye movements in tachistoscopic perception. *Canadian Journal of Psychology*, 1961, 15, 220–225.

CHOUDHURY, B. P., WHITTERIDGE, D., & WILSON, M. E. The function of the callosal connections of the visual cortex. *Quarterly Journal of Experimental Physiology*, 1965, 50, 214–219.

CLARKE, J. C. Response asymmetry, stimulus control and the mirror-image reversal phenomenon: An operant analysis. Unpublished master's thesis. University of Auckland, 1969.

CORBALLIS, M. C., & BEALE, I. L. Interocular transfer following simultaneous discrimination of mirror-image stimuli. *Psychonomic Science,* 1967, 9, 605–606.

CORBALLIS, M. C., & BEALE, I. L. Monocular discrimination of mirror-image obliques by pigeons: Evidence for lateralized stimulus control. *Animal Behavior,* 1970, in press.

DEUTSCH, J. A. A theory of shape recognition. *British Journal of Psychology,* 1955, 46, 30–37.

DODWELL, P. C. Shape recognition in rats. *British Journal of Psychology,* 1957, 48, 221–229.

DOWNER, J. L., deC. Interhemispheric integration in the visual system. In V. B. Mountcastle (Ed.), *Interhemispheric relations and cerebral dominance.* Baltimore: Johns Hopkins Press, 1962.

ETTLINGER, G., & ELITHORN, A. Transfer between the hands of a mirror-image tactile shape discrimination. *Nature,* 1962, 194, 1101.

FRITSCH, V. *Left and right in science and life.* London: Barrie & Rockcliff, 1968.

GARDNER, M. *The ambidextrous universe.* New York: Basic Books, 1964.

GAZZANIGA, M. S. Cerebral dominance and lateral specialization. Paper presented at the meeting of the American Psychological Association, San Francisco, September 1968.

GAZZANIGA, M. S., & SPERRY, R. W. Language after section of the cerebral commissures. *Brain,* 1967, 90, 131–148.

GRAFSTEIN, B. Organization of callosal connections in suprasylvian gyrus of cat. *Journal of Neurophysiology,* 1959, 22, 504–515.

GRINDLEY, G. C. The formation of a simple habit in guinea pigs. *British Journal of Psychology,* 1932, 23, 127–147.

HEBB, D. O. *Organization of behavior.* New York: Wiley, 1949.

HEBB, D. O. The semiautonomous process: Its nature and nurture. *American Psychologist,* 1963, 18, 16–27.

HODOS, W., & CAMPBELL, C. B. G. *Scala naturae:* Why there is no theory in comparative psychology. *Psychological Review,* 1969, 76, 337–350.

HUBEL, D. H., & WIESEL, T. N. Receptive fields, binocular interaction, and functional architecture in the cat's visual cortex. *Journal of Physiology,* 1962, 160, 106–123.

HUBEL, D. H., & WIESEL, T. N. Cortical and callosal connections concerned with the vertical meridian of visual fields in the cat. *Journal of Neurophysiology,* 1967, 30, 1561–1573.

HUIZINGA, E., & VAN DER MEULEN, P. Vestibulary rotatory and optokinetic reactions in the pigeon. *Annals of Otology, Rhinology and Laryngology,* 1951, 60, 928–948.

INGLE, D. Two visual mechanisms underlying the behavior of fish. *Psychologische Forschung,* 1967, 31, 44–51.

JEFFREY, W. E. Variables in early discrimination learning: I. Motor responses in the training of a left-right discrimination. *Child Development,* 1958, 29, 269–275.

KONORSKI, J. On the mechanism of instrumental conditioning. In, *Proceedings of the 17th international congress of psychology.* Amsterdam: North Holland Publishing, 1964.

LASHLEY, K. S. The mechanism of vision, XV. Preliminary studies of the rat's capacity for detailed vision. *Journal of General Psychology,* 1938, 18, 123–193.

MACH, E. *Popular scientific lectures.* Chicago: Open Court Publishing House, 1894.

MACH, E. *The analysis of sensations.* New York: Dover, 1959. (Originally published, 1900.)

MACKINTOSH, J., & SUTHERLAND, N. S. Visual discrimination by the goldfish: The orientation of rectangles. *Animal Behavior,* 1963, 11, 135–141.

MAKITA, K. The rarity of reading disability in Japanese children. *American Journal of Orthopsychiatry,* 1968, 38, 599–614.

MELLO, N. K. Interhemispheric reversal of mirror-image oblique lines after monocular training in pigeons. *Science,* 1965, 148, 252–254.

MELLO, N. K. Concerning the interhemisphere transfer of mirror-image oblique lines after monocular training in pigeons. *Physiology and Behavior,* 1966, 1, 293–300. (a)

MELLO, N. K. Interocular generalization: A study of mirror-image reversal following monocular training in pigeons. *Journal of the Experimental Analysis of Behavior,* 1966, 9, 11–16. (b)

MELLO, N. K. The effect of unilateral lesions of the optic tectum on interhemispheric transfer of monocularly trained color and pattern discrimination in pigeon. *Physiology and Behavior,* 1968, 3, 725–734.

MILLIKAN, C. H., & DARLEY, F. L. (Eds.) *Brain mechanisms underlying speech and language.* New York: Grune & Stratton, 1967.

MORRELL, P. Information storage in nerve cells. In W. S. Fields & W. Abbott (Eds.), *Information storage and neural control.* Springfield, Ill.: Charles C Thomas, 1963.

MOUNTCASTLE, V. B. (Ed.) *Interhemispheric relations and cerebral dominance.* Baltimore: Johns Hopkins Press, 1962.

MYERS, R. E. Corpus callosum and interhemispheric communication: Enduring memory effects. *Federal Proceedings,* 1957, 16, 92.

MYERS, R. E. Commissural connections between occipital lobes of the monkey. *Journal of Comparative Neurology,* 1962, 118, 1–16.

NISSEN, H. W., & McCULLOCH, T. L. Equated and non-equated stimulus conditions in discrimination learning by chimpanzees: I. Comparison with unlimited response. *Journal of Comparative Psychology,* 1937, 23, 165–189.

NOBLE, J. Mirror-images and the forebrain commissures of the monkey. *Nature,* 1966, **211,** 1263–1265.

NOBLE, J. Paradoxical interocular transfer of mirror-image discrimination in the optic chiasm sectioned monkey. *Brain Research,* 1968, **10,** 127–151.

OVER, R. Detection and recognition measures of shape discrimination. *Nature,* 1967, **214,** 1272–1273.

OVER, R., & OVER, J. Detection and recognition of mirror-image obliques by young children. *Journal of Comparative and Physiological Psychology,* 1967, **64,** 467–470.

PAVLOV, I. P. *Conditioned reflexes.* London: Oxford University Press, 1927.

RAY, O. S., & EMLEY, G. Time factors in interhemispheric transfer of learning. *Science,* 1964, **144,** 76–78.

RAY, O. S., & EMLEY, G. Interhemispheric transfer of learning. *Life Sciences,* 1965, **4,** 823–826.

RESTLE, F. Discrimination of cues in mazes: A resolution of the "place-vs.-response" question. *Psychological Review,* 1957, **64,** 217–228.

RIOPELLE, A. J., ITOIGAWA, N., RAHM, V., & DRAPER, W. A. Discrimination of mirror-image patterns by rhesus monkeys. *Perceptual and Motor Skills,* 1964, **19,** 383–389.

RUDEL, R. G., & TEUBER, H. L. Discrimination of direction of line in children. *Journal of Comparative and Physiological Psychology,* 1963, **56,** 892–898.

SPERRY, R. W. Some general aspects of interhemispheric integration. In V. B. Mountcastle (Ed.), *Interhemispheric relations and cerebral dominance.* Baltimore: Johns Hopkins Press, 1962.

STIER, E. *Untersuchangen uber Linkshandigkeit.* Jena: G. Fischer, 1911. Cited by G. von Bonin, Anatomical asymmetries of the cerebral hemispheres. In V. B. Mountcastle (Ed.), *Interhemispheric relations and cerebral dominance* Baltimore: Johns Hopkins Press, 1962. P. 1.

SUTHERLAND, N. S. Visual discrimination of orientation and shape by Octopus. *Nature,* 1957, **179,** 11–13.

SUTHERLAND, N. S. Visual discrimination of shape by *Octopus:* Mirror images. *British Journal of Psychology,* 1960, **51,** 9–18.

SUTHERLAND, N. S. Cat's ability to discriminate oblique rectangles. *Science,* 1963, **139,** 209–210.

TREVARTHEN, C. B. Manipulative strategies of baboons and the origins of cerebral asymmetry. In M. Kinsbourne (Ed.), *Hemisphere asymmetry of function.* London: Tavistock, 1970, in press.

TSCHIRGI, R. D. Spatial perception and central nervous system symmetry. *Arquivos de Neuropsiquiatria,* 1958, **16,** 364–366.

WALK, R. D. Monocular compared to binocular depth perception in human infants. *Science,* 1968, **162,** 473–475.

WEYL, H. *Symmetry.* Princeton, N. J.: Princeton University Press, 1953.

WHITTERIDGE, D. Area 18 and the vertical meridian of the visual field. In E. G. Ettlinger (Ed.), *Functions of the Corpus Callosum.* (Ciba Foundation Study Group No. 20) London: Churchill, 1965.

YOUNG, J. Z. Why do we have two brains? In V. B. Mountcastle (Ed.), *Interhemispheric relations and cerebral dominance.* Baltimore: Johns Hopkins Press, 1962.

LATERAL DOMINANCE AND RIGHT-LEFT
AWARENESS IN NORMAL CHILDREN [1]

LILLIAN BELMONT *and* HERBERT G. BIRCH   [2]

One of the normal patterns of developmental change consists in the establishment of hand preferences for skilled manual activities. In addition, the development of such consistent preferences in the majority of individuals bears a systematic relation to the establishment of preponderant usage in other bilaterally represented functions such as vision and lower limb utilization. Knowledge of the details of the development of such preferences in normal children is of especial importance because of the emphasis which has been placed upon the significance of this feature of development for normal educational functioning (8, 9), language and reading functions (11), and personality patterning (3).

Despite the existence of a large body of normative evidence on lateralization (9), little information is available as to the ages at which various aspects of lateralization come to be established. A qualitative approach to this problem was made in an early study by Gesell and Ames (6), and evidence for some specific ages has been reported by Harris for lateral domi-

[1] This investigation was supported by Grant B-3362 of the National Institutes of Health, National Institute of Neurological Diseases and Blindness, and the Association for the Aid of Crippled Children.

[2] The authors wish to express their gratitude to Juliet Bortner, who participated in the collection of data, and to the West Hempstead School District, which made it possible to conduct this and other studies in their schools.

CHILD DEVELOPMENT, 1963, Vol. 34, pp. 257-270.

nance (8) and by Benton (1) for right-left discrimination. However, both these age specific analyses have covered a restricted age range.

A further complication preventing a clear understanding of the development of laterality is that different methods have been used for determining lateral dominance. Consequently, it is difficult to determine whether reported differences are the result of the differences in the samples of children tested or of the test methods used for determining dominance. In addition, since it has been claimed by many (9) that preferential hand usage in children may be significantly affected by cultural milieu and contemporary styles in the amount of pressure applied to children to cause them to use the right hand, consideration at the present time must necessarily be based on evidence derived from children who have been raised in the current atmosphere of childrearing practices. The problems arising from the above considerations can be resolved by obtaining contemporary data on age specificities in the establishment of lateral dominance.

A second issue with which we have been concerned is the question of right-left awareness. The ability to make reliable right-left discriminations both with reference to the child's own body and to the surrounding environment represents another aspect of lateralized functioning which follows a recognizable developmental course (12), and disturbance in this area has been related to developmental dysfunctions in a manner very similar to that ascribed to preference in lateral usage (10, 8). Although information is available indicating a small positive relation between discriminative function and handedness (2), little information is available concerning the relation, if any, between right-left discrimination and a fuller spectrum of preferential usage involved in eyedness and eye-hand preferences. These questions could be answered by obtaining contemporary information on the development of right-left discrimination in the same children in whom the general development of lateral dominance was being studied.

The present study, therefore, is concerned with the analysis of age-specificity in preferential lateral usage, the development of right-left awareness, and the relation between the two sets of functions in normal children of school age.

METHOD

Subjects

The subjects studied were 148 children drawn from a suburban elementary school for intellectually normal children. The class placement of children ranged from kindergarten through sixth grade with ages from 5 years, 3 months, to 12 years, 5 months. The number of boys was equal to the number of girls and the two sexes were insignificantly different in IQ, grade placement, and age. Selection from the whole school population was made from a master list containing the names of children from kindergarten through sixth grade whose parents had given permission for testing. Within this list, selection at each grade level was on a random basis. Otis Quick-Scoring Tests of Mental Ability were available for all children from the third grade level through the sixth grade. The parents of the children were either in skilled or professional occupations and of middle class socioeconomic standing. As may be seen from Table 1, in which salient characteristics of the sample are presented, the mean IQ was significantly above the general population average, as would be expected on the basis of the socioeconomic groups to which the families of the children belonged.

TABLE 1

AGE, SEX, AND IQ OF SUBJECTS

		C A		I Q *	
	N	Mean	SD	Mean	SD
Male	74	8-3	2-0	119.8	10.4
Female	74	8-2	2-0	120.2	10.3
Total	148	8-2	2-0	120.0	10.3

* IQ (Otis Quick-Scoring Test of Mental Ability) available for 65 subjects (32 boys; 33 girls) 8 years and older who were routinely tested in school.

Procedure

All children were taken from the classroom by the examiner and tested individually. Lateral dominance was studied first and was followed by the testing of right-left awareness. All testing was conducted in a single session.

Hand preference. Lateral preference was tested for hand, eye, and foot. The subjects were required to respond in pantomime to hand preference items. The following four items were used:

> a. *Ball throwing.* The experimenter says, "This is how I throw a ball." (demonstrates) "Now let me see you throw a ball."
>
> b. *Turning door knob.* The experimenter says, "I turn a door knob this way." (demonstrates) "Let me see how you turn a door knob."
>
> c. *Scissor cutting.* The experimenter says, "I cut with scissors this way." (demonstrates) "Let me see how you do it."
>
> d. *Writing.* The experimenter says, "When I write with a pencil, I move my hand this way." (demonstrates) "Let me see how you move your hand with a pencil when you write."

The hand used by the child for each of these pantomime activities was recorded.

Eye preference. In determining eyedness, three tasks were used, a kaleidoscope, a toy rifle, and a square of paper with a ½-in. square hole in the center.

a. *Kaleidoscope.* The child was handed the kaleidoscope and told, "Look through this."

b. *Rifle sighting.* The experimenter handed the child the toy rifle and asked, "Do you know how to aim a rifle?" If the child said "Yes," he was asked to do so. If the child said "No," he was told to "close one eye, look through the hole, hold it on your shoulder and make believe you are going to shoot."

c. *Paper with hole.* E handed the child a 6-in. square of paper with a ½-in. square hole in the center. The child was told, "Look at me through this hole."

The eye which was used was noted for each task.

Foot preference. Foot preference was determined by studying kicking. The experimenter placed a ball 5 in. in diameter on a plastic wedge which was located on the floor. The child was instructed to "kick the ball." After the spontaneous foot usage, the examiner instructed the child to kick the ball with the other foot. Examiner noted the foot first used and which kick was more skillfully executed. When there was no clear-cut difference between the two feet in level of skill, the child was asked, "Which foot do you like to kick with better?"

Rating criteria for lateral dominance: Handedness was scored as "right" if all four tasks were mimicked with the right hand; "left" if all four tasks were done with the left hand; "mixed" if in the series of four tasks there was any inconsistency in hand usage.

The subject was judged as right- or left-eyed if he used the given eye consistently on all three of the tasks. The subject was rated "mixed" if on any occasion he was inconsistent in eye usage.

The foot spontaneously chosen for first kick was scored as the preferred foot. If the preferred foot was superior in its performance to the nonpreferred one, preference and dominance were the same. If the nonpreferred foot functioned better, dominance was rated as mixed. Following Harris' standards (7), footedness was rated as "mixed" if performance on both feet was equally skilled.

Awareness of right-left relations. In order to test the child's ability to make right-left discriminations on own body parts, two tests were used. One was a three-item test in which the following questions were asked: 1. Raise your right hand. 2. Touch your left ear. 3. Point to your right eye. The other test had four items: 1. Show me your right hand. 2. Now show me your left hand. 3. Show me your right leg. 4. Now show me your left leg. These last four items form part of the Piaget schedule.

In addition, each subject was asked to respond to a series of other questions derived from Piaget (12) concerning awareness of right-left relations on other than own body. The tasks designed by Piaget include the identification of lateralization on the body of the examiner facing the child, as well as the degree to which awareness of right-left object relations exists. The conditions and questions involved in these tasks are indicated below.

All responses were recorded, and any item was scored as correct if all of its component parts were answered appropriately.

Right-Left Awareness Items (Piaget)

1. Show me your right hand. _____ Now show me your left hand. _____
   Show me your right leg. _____ Now show me your left leg. _____

2. (E sits opposite S)   Show me my right hand. _____
   Now my left. _____   Show me my right leg. _____
   Now my left leg. _____

3. (Place coin on table left of a pencil in relation to S.)
   Is the pencil to the right or to the left? _____
   And the penny—is it to the right or to the left? _____
   (Have S go around to the opposite side of table and repeat questions.)
   Is the pencil to the right or to the left? _____
   And the penny—it it to the right or to the left? _____

4. (S is opposite E; E has a coin in right hand and a bracelet [or watch] on left arm.) You see this penny. Have I got it in my right hand or in my left? _____   And the bracelet. Is it on my right arm or my left? _____

5. (S is opposite three objects in a row: a pencil to the left, a key in the middle, and a coin to the right.)
   Is the pencil to the left or to the right of the key? _____
   Is the pencil to the left or to the right of the penny? _____
   Is the key to the left or to the right of the penny? _____
   Is the key to the left or to the right of the pencil? _____
   Is the penny to the left or to the right of the pencil? _____
   Is the penny to the left or to the right of the key? _____

A separate analysis was made of all questions relating to right-left discrimination of the parts of the child's own body.

RESULTS

Lateral Dominance

The over-all results on lateralization of hand, eye, and foot functioning, as well as hand-eye interrelations, in our sample of children are presented in Tables 2 and 3. As may be seen from Table 2, the children as a whole are predominantly right-handed (76 per cent), 10 per cent are left-handed, and 14 per cent have handedness which is rated as "mixed." The mixed group is composed of 11 subjects who were preponderantly right-handed in their responses, five subjects who were preponderantly left-handed, and five who exhibited equal right- and left-handed preference. Since the largest number of subjects in the mixed group were in the younger ages, the subjects in the mixed category are a composite of stably mixed individuals and of younger children in whom hand preference has not yet been fully established. If the criterion is lowered and the children who show only single instances of inconsistency in hand preference are included in the dominant group, then the percentages of right-handed and left-handed children in-

TABLE 2

LATERALITY PREFERENCES FOR THE GROUP OF NORMAL CHILDREN

Category	Totals N=148	AGE-SPECIFIC PERCENTAGES *						
		5-3 to 5-11 N=23	6-0 to 6-11 N=25	7-0 to 7-11 N=28	8-0 to 8-11 N=20	9-0 to 9-11 N=17	10-0 to 10-11 N=14	11-0 to 11-11 N=18
Handedness								
Right	113 (76%)	87	60	75	75	82	79	83
Left	14 (10%)	5	12	4	10	12	21	6
Mixed ...	21 (14%)	9	28	21	15	6	0	11
Eyedness								
Right	78 (53%)	44	52	43	60	41	57	78
Left	31 (21%)	31	20	21	15	24	29	6
Mixed ...	39 (26%)	26	28	36	25	35	14	17
Footedness								
Right	125 (85%)	83	88	89	80	88	79	83
Left	17 (12%)	9	8	7	15	12	21	11
Mixed ...	6 (4%)	9	4	4	5	0	0	6
Hand-Eye								
Consistent	71 (48%)	39	36	36	50	41	78	67
Crossed ..	24 (16%)	31	16	14	15	24	8	6
Mixed ...	53 (36%)	31	48	50	35	35	14	28

* Age 12 omitted because of small N.

crease at the expense of the mixed group. We then find that 13 per cent exhibit left preference, 84 per cent right preference, and 3 per cent remain as truly mixed. The figure of 13 per cent left-handed is higher than the percentage usually reported in the general population and may be a reflection of some relaxation in contemporary pressures used in the social induction of hand usage in children.

On the basis of our findings, eye preference does not exhibit the same degree of lateralization as does handedness. More than 25 per cent of the children in the age range studied failed to exhibit clear-cut preferential use of one eye and so were rated as mixed. Of the remaining children, 53 per cent are consistently right-eyed and 21 per cent show left eye preference. The age specificity of both eye and hand preference will be considered below.

Of all our findings, the one which exhibits the most clear-cut and earliest established preference in usage is footedness. Over 95 per cent of the children show clear-cut lateral dominance in foot usage. Only 4 per cent showed

TABLE 3

AGE DIFFERENCES IN LATERALITY PREFERENCES

	5-3 to 5-11	6-0 to 6-11	7-0 to 7-11	8-0 to 8-11	9-0 to 9-11	10-0 to 10-11	11-0 to 11-11	12-0 to 12-5	χ^2	df	p[†]
Handedness											
Right and Left	39		39			49					
Mixed	9		9			3			4.71	2	< .05
Eyedness											
Right and Left	17	18	18	15	11	12	18				
Mixed	6	7	10	5	6	2	3		4.58	6	< .30
Footedness											
Right and Left	45		46		31		20				
Mixed	3		2		0		1				ns
Hand-Eye											
Consistent	9	9	10	10	7	11	12	3			
Crossed and Mixed	14	16	18	10	10	3	6	0	15.45	7	< .02

[*] Because of the nature of the distributions, it was at times necessary to combine age groups to satisfy the requirements for the use of the chi square test.

[†] One-tailed test because of directional nature of hypothesis.

mixed foot dominance. Within the age range considered no significant difference in degree of foot lateralization is to be found on an age-specific basis (Table 3). Thus, by the time the children are in the sixth year of life, preferential foot utilization has already been clearly established. For this reason, an age-specific consideration of footedness is not possible in our sample and would require the study of younger children.

The age specificity of hand and eye preferences may be determined from an inspection of Tables 2 and 3. Table 2 presents our first order data in terms of age-specific percentages. Table 3 presents these data in terms of the actual number of cases at various age categories for statistical tests of significance. It will be noted in Table 3 that right and left preferences are treated as a single variable since we are interested in the developmental course of consistent preferential usage as opposed to mixed usage, rather than in either right or left usage as such. Because of the nature of the distributions, it was at times necessary to combine age groups to satisfy the requirements for the use of the chi square test.

It is apparent from Table 2 that mixed handedness is most pronounced in the 6-, 7-, and 8-year-old subjects, but is not evident in the 5-year-old group. It can be seen from the table that mixed handedness characterizes the younger children far more frequently than it does the older ones. These age differences in hand usage are significant at the .05 level of confidence (Table 3). As may be seen from Table 2, the tenth year of life appears to be the one at which a high level of consistency in preferential hand usage becomes established. At this age, the developmental curve appears to become asymptotic to the age base. When the handedness of children below 9 years was contrasted with the handedness above this age, there was a statistically significant difference ($\chi^2 = 3.66$; $df = 1$; $p < .03$, one-tailed) between the two age groups. This suggests that for populations similar to the one studied age 9 may represent a useful indicator for the existence of reliably established preferential hand usage, when our criterion of 100 per cent consistency in the four handedness tasks is employed.

A similar trend may be found in the establishment of clear-cut preferences in monocular eye usage (Table 2). The level of mixed eyedness is greater in the younger than in the older age groups. While the age differences in eyedness do not achieve an acceptable level of statistical significance (Table 3), an examination of the individual cells does appear to show an increase in right and left eyedness from age 10. When the data were analyzed using age 10 as a cut-off point, statistically significant differences were found between the younger and older children ($\chi^2 = 2.67$; $df = 1$; $p < .05$, one-tailed). In large part, this results from the fact that there was a larger proportion of mixed eyedness in the group below 10 years.

The relation of preferential hand to preferential eye usage is also considered in Table 2. As may be seen, approximately one half of the total group exhibits ipsilateral preferences. The other half of the group shows a pattern of inconsistency in preferential lateral usage. This is expressed either through the contralateral use of hand and eye or as the ill-established dominance in either one of these functions. In terms of the age specificity of eye-hand relations, it may be seen that there is a general tendency for ipsilateral utilization of hand and eye to increase with age. Conversely, as the children grow older a smaller proportion of individuals exhibit mixed or cross hand-eye usage. As may be seen in Table 3, hand-eye relations show highly significant age differences ($\chi^2 = 15.45$; $p < .02$), which are also reflected in a reliable difference in functioning in children below and above age 10 ($\chi^2 = 11.37$; $df = 1$; $p < .001$). Thus, by the age of 10, eye-hand dominance interrelations appear to be reliably stabilized, and children above this age are significantly more ipsilateral.

Since there have been repeated reports (4, 9) that left-handedness and confusion in lateralization occur more frequently in boys than in girls, our data were examined for sex differences in preferential hand usage. These findings are summarized in Table 4. In our group of normal children no significant sex differences in handedness were found. On an absolute basis the girls showed somewhat more of a tendency (not statistically significant) to be left- or mixed-handed than did the boys. These findings agree

TABLE 4

HAND PREFERENCES IN BOYS AND GIRLS

	Right	Left	Mixed
Boys ($N=74$)	59 (80%)	6 (8%)	9 (12%)
Girls ($N=74$)	54 (73%)	8 (11%)	12 (16%)

with other current reports (5, 8) in which no reliable sex differences in handedness were found.

Right-Left Awareness

The second set of issues with which we have been concerned in the present investigation is the awareness of right-left relations. The study of this awareness involved at least two general features. The first of these was awareness by the child of the lateralization of the parts of his own body. The second concerned awareness of lateral placement of objects in the environment including parts of other individuals located at 180 degrees to the child.

In Tables 5 and 6 our findings on the age-specific awareness of left-right relations on own body are considered. As may be seen from these tables, failures, when they occur, were to be found in the younger age groups. These age differences are statistically significant. In the 5- and 6-year-olds, there was a larger percentage of children who failed one or more of the seven questions (consisting of three of our own items plus four of Piaget's items), which tapped ability to distinguish left from right on own body

TABLE 5

AGE-SPECIFIC PERCENTAGES OF ACCURACY IN RIGHT-LEFT
DISCRIMINATION OF OWN BODY PARTS

Age	N	Percentage Passed All Questions	Percentage Failed a Given No. of Questions						
			1	2	3	4	5	6	7
5-3 to 5-11	23	70	13	9	0	0	4	0	4
6-0 to 6-11	25	68	4	12	4	12	0	0	0
7-0 to 7-11	28	89	4	0	4	4	0	0	0
8-0 to 8-11	20	95	0	0	5	0	0	0	0
9-0 to 9-11	17	94	6	0	0	0	0	0	0
10-0 to 10-11	14	100	0	0	0	0	0	0	0
11-0 to 11-11	18	100	0	0	0	0	0	0	0
12-0 to 12- 5	3	100	0	0	0	0	0	0	0

TABLE 6

AGE DIFFERENCES IN ACCURACY OF RIGHT-LEFT DISCRIMINATION OF OWN BODY PARTS

| | A G E   R A N G E S | | | χ^2 | df | p |
	5-3 to 6-11	7-0 to 8-11	9-0 to 12-5			
Passed all questions.......	33	44	51			
Failed one or more questions	15	4	1	19.91	2	.001

parts. Rarely were these children characterized by complete failure to distinguish left from right but rather by an occasional confusion. However, in the present sample even the youngest children were frequently able to be entirely correct in their ability to distinguish left and right on their own bodies.

As may be seen from an inspection of Table 5, 95 per cent of the children above 7 years of age make correct responses to all seven questions concerned with the lateralization of their own body parts. In contrast, only 69 per cent of the children below 7 years of age in our sample correctly answered all questions regarding own body parts. (The significance of the difference in performance between children under 7 and those over this age is at the .001 level of confidence.) It is of interest to note that the accuracy of right-left awareness of own body parts antedates the clear-cut establishment of hand preference by 2 years and of eyedness and eye-hand consistency by 3 years.

Table 7 presents a comparison of our findings on the ages at which the subjects passed the various items on the Piaget schedule of awareness of right

TABLE 7

COMPARISON OF GROUP WITH PIAGET AGE NORMS ON LEFT-RIGHT CONCEPTIONS

| | ITEM No. PASSED* | |
	Our Sample	Piaget Norms
Age 5	1	1
Age 6	1	1
Age 7	1, 3, 4	1, 3
Age 8	1, 2, 3, 4	1, 2, 3, 4
Age 9	1, 2, 3, 4	1, 2, 3, 4
Age 10	1, 2, 3, 4	1, 2, 3, 4
Age 11	1, 2, 3, 4, 5†	1, 2, 3, 4, 5

* 75 per cent or more of group passed item.
† 72 per cent of group passed.

41

and left with those that he has reported (12). We followed Piaget's procedure and used 75 per cent of the children for any age correct on an item as the criterion for considering an item passed by this age group. Using this criterion, we found that there was a remarkable agreement in the development of right-left conceptions in our group and in his. The only apparent discrepancies were that at age 7 our group was able to distinguish the lateral placement of objects on another person's body (item 4) whereas Piaget's group could not. The findings reported in Table 7 indicate that by age 7 our group is able successfully to distinguish right-left relations on own body parts and on another person's body placed at 180 degrees to him. However, the ability to distinguish object lateralization in the environment did not stabilize until age 11 (item 5). It should be noted that the criterion for passing is less stringent in this analysis than in the one presented in Table 5.

Right-left awareness was studied in relation to a variety of other factors. No consistent relation was found between the level of performance on items of right-left awareness and any other factor of lateral preference studied (chi square analysis by age). There were no significant sex differences in level of performance. Grade placement was not related in any reliable fashion to right-left awareness, although there was some tendency for the children of the same chronological age level who were in higher grades (e.g., 7-year-olds placed in grade 2 rather than 1) to function somewhat better than did their age mates. There were no reliable differences in performance when right-left awareness was related to IQ within the range represented in our sample.

DISCUSSION

The findings of the present study will be considered in connection with three issues: (a) age specificity in the development of lateralization; (b) the relation between right-left discrimination and lateralization of function; and (c) the implications of age specificity in lateralization and right-left discrimination for the etiology of reading disability.

The question of age specificity in the development of lateralization has received too scant attention. An indication of the age span within which laterality in function becomes stabilized is of especial importance if lateralization is to be used as one of the diagnostic indicators of developmental abnormality in children. An early attempt at age-specific treatment may be found in the report of Gesell and Ames (6) who present some qualitative findings. Although their qualitative findings are suggestive, they do not provide any firm statistical basis for deciding when stable lateral preference is to be expected in the normally developing child. In more recent reports, the studies by Harris (8) and Benton (1) provide some additional data on age-specific functioning.

Although Harris has presented data on the distribution of lateral dominance in hand, eye, and foot usage for two age groups, 7- and 9-year-olds, our findings suggest that these ages do not provide the most significant points for analysis of the developmental course of lateralization. On the basis of our analysis of the ages at which functions become stabilized in the present sample, we would differentiate between ambilaterality in handedness which occurs before age 9 and that which occurs after that time, since we found a critical break at this age in the number of children in the present sample who exhibited mixed handedness. In addition, our findings indicate that the development of preferential handedness is by no means a continuously developing function since the level of consistent preferential usage exhibited by our 5-year-old kindergarten group is not again achieved until the age of 9 years. This finding is in general agreement with the observation of Gesell and Ames that preferential hand usage is subject to peaks and troughs on an age-specific basis. It would be of considerable interest to explore the reorganizational changes in functioning that underlie these changes in preference.

In considering correspondence between eye and hand usage, we found that a chronological age of 10 was modal for the normal establishment of ipsilaterality. Prior to this age, less than half of the children exhibited consistent ipsilateral hand-eye usage. Since normal children below the age of 9 show evidences of both incomplete lateral preference and hand-eye ambilaterality until the age of 10, the usefulness of such findings for the definition of developmental pathology in younger age groups is of questionable value. If, however, consistent lateral preference and ipsilateral usage of hand and eye do not develop in subsequent years, the findings may be viewed as suggestive of developmental aberration, since it may be indicative of a lag in normal developmental function.

Benton (1) presents data on normative aspects of right-left discrimination in terms of norms for ages 6 through 9. Because of the limitation in the age range he has studied, he has stated that "it is not possible to specify the exact age at which the level of average adult performance is achieved" (1, p. 27) since his data on the performances of children above 9 are incomplete. However, it is clear from his formulation that age specificity in this function is a problem which he believes to be of major importance. On the basis of our data on bright normal children from a middle class background, the age of 7 appears to be critical for the development of the ability to distinguish left and right in relation to one's own body parts. Subsequent to this age, up to the age of 12, little significant improvement in this ability takes place, and from age 10 onward all children studied pass all questions asked. When the demand was shifted from own body parts to objects in the external environment, fully accurate right-left awareness was not stabilized in ages below the 11-year-old group.

In our findings no simple relation was found to exist between the establishment of lateral preference in hand usage and the development of the ability to discriminate right from left. Children of a given age in whom preferential hand usage was clearly established did not differ significantly in their ability to distinguish right from left from children of the same age in whom preferential hand usage had not yet come to be firmly established. Conversely, at a given age the ability accurately to discriminate right from left did not permit the prediction of preferential lateralization in hand usage. When considered age specifically, it was found that accurate right-left discrimination, at least of own body parts, preceded the stabilization of lateral hand preference by approximately two years.

Considerable interest attaches to the fact that discrimination of right and left antedates the development of consistent lateral hand usage. It makes it highly improbable that the development of right-left awareness (which develops earlier) is dependent upon consistent lateralization of hand usage (which occurs two years later). A more parsimonious interpretation would view the two functions as independent aspects of development. If this position is taken, the implications that have been drawn between the development of hand preference and reading disability must be reassessed.

Numerous workers (8, 11) have reported a relation between reading disability and lag in lateralization in function. At times there has even been the implication, as Benton has noted, that such delay in maturation of lateral dominance may be etiologically related to reading dysfunction because of the frequently expressed assumption that right-left discrimination, necessary in the reading task, requires preferential lateral hand usage for its establishment. An age-specific analysis of both right-left discrimination and lateralization of functions raises questions about the validity of this chain of reasoning. Our own data indicate that the establishment of reliable right-left discrimination antedates by several years the development of consistent lateralized preferences in hand usage. An even greater lag exists between preferential eye dominance and right-left discriminative capacity. It is therefore most unlikely that visual discrimination and awareness of the difference of right from left is dependent upon preferential hand or eye usage. It is far more likely that developmental lag in lateralization and evidence of reading disability are independent manifestations of a more general underlying disturbance in neurological organization and are not etiologically related to one another. A similar line of reasoning can be applied to those studies in which lags in the establishment of lateral dominance have been related to emotional and personality disorders (3).

Summary

Lateral preferences in hand, eye, and foot usage and awareness of right-left relations were examined in 148 bright normal children from a suburban school system. It was found that clear-cut establishment of hand and eye preferences could be analyzed on an age-specific basis and that ambilaterality more frequently characterized the younger age groups. Discrimination of right-left relations also followed a developmental course with all aspects of discrimination, including own body parts, other person opposite the subject, and object relations in the environment, tending to become stabilized at age 11. Right-left discrimination of own body parts is clearly stabilized at age 7, two years prior to the establishment of consistent handedness and three years prior to the stabilization of eyedness and eye-hand preferences. The presence of deviancy in these two functions in younger children was considered to be of questionable diagnostic value. The appearance of right-left discrimination on own body parts at an earlier age than the clear-cut establishment of handedness suggests that these two functions are independent. This was discussed in relation to the question of the etiology of reading disability.

REFERENCES

1. BENTON, A. L. *Right-left discrimination and finger localization.* Hoeber-Harper, 1959.
2. BENTON, A. L., & MENEFEE, F. L. Handedness and right-left discrimination. *Child Develpm.*, 1957, 28, 237-242.
3. BLAU, A. *The master hand: a study of the origin and meaning of right and left sidedness and its relation to personality and language.* Amer. Orthopsychiat. Ass., 1946.
4. BRAIN, R. W. Speech and handedness. *Lancet*, 1945, 2, 837-842.
5. FALEK, A. Handedness: a family study. *Amer. J. hum. Genet.*, 1959, 11, 52-62.
6. GESELL, A., & AMES, L. B. The development of handedness. *J. genet. Psychol.*, 1947, 70, 155-175.
7. HARRIS, A. J. *Harris Tests of Lateral Dominance.* (Manual, 3rd Ed.) Psychol. Corp., 1947.
8. HARRIS, A. J. Lateral dominance, directional confusion, and reading disability. *J. Psychol.*, 1957, 44, 283-294.
9. HILDRETH, G. The development and training of hand dominance. *J. genet. Psychol.*, 1949, 75, 197-275; 1950, 76, 39-144.
10. KENNARD, M. A. Value of equivocal signs in neurologic diagnosis. *Neurology*, 1960, 10, 753-764.
11. ORTON, S. T. *Reading, writing and speech problems in children.* Norton, 1937.
12. PIAGET, J. *Judgment and reasoning in the child.* Kegan Paul, 1928.

DEVELOPMENT OF THE SENSE OF BALANCE IN SCHOOL CHILDREN*

GERALD W. CRON
N. H. PRONKO

THE YEAR old infant finds it difficult or impossible to maintain his balance. The two year old does much better. Does his "sense of balance" continue to improve with age? When does improvement cease? Are there sex differences in this ability to maintain equilibrium? This study was undertaken with the purpose of answering such questions as a basis for further research.

Procedure

Subjects consisted of 501 children òn fourteen of the summer playgrounds supervised by the Parks Department, City of Wichita. There were 322 boys and 179 girls, ranging in age from 4 to 15 years.

The balance board is a "two-by-four" twelve feet long, supported on edge four inches from either end, two inches from the ground. Having no middle support, it sags and sways somewhat, requiring compensatory movements by the walker.

The children were told that this was a way to test their ability to balance, like a circus tight rope walker. The examiner demonstrated by walking the board and explained the scoring as follows: "Each child gets three trials at walking the board. If he steps off the board before walking the length of it, that constitues a trial and he scores a "0". If he manages to walk the length of the board he scores a "1". If he makes a "roundtrip" without stepping off, he scores a "2". Thus, a perfect score for the three trials is "6".

At twelve of the playgrounds the balance board was placed so that all children had access to it. The examiner was there at all times and explained the procedure. Those who wished tried the experiment. Most of the children were interested and volunteered. Onlookers were kept about ten feet from the board. Playground directors were cooperative. There was little, if any, bantering.

At two of the playgrounds the balance board was put into a room and children were tested one at a time. In this case the explanation was made to each child individually. This variation in procedure did not radically upset our

*The authors wish to express their appreciation for the cooperation of Mr. Pat Haggerty and Mr. Tom Allen of the Parks Department, City of Wichita, Kansas. They also appreciate the help of the directors of fourteen of the summer playgrounds and of over five hundred children who took part in the experiment.

JOURNAL OF EDUCATIONAL RESEARCH, 1957, Vol. 51, pp. 33-37.

norms, a fact indicated by the similarity of our results under these two conditions and with those of Sloan discussed below, but it did suggest some f u r -
ther research possibilities.

Results and Discussion

Inspection of Table I shows that the ability of children to walk the balance
board increases with age from the 4-6 group (average score 0.3) to the 11-12
year group (average score 3.3). It then levels off and shows a slight decline
in the 12-15 year group. All of the youngest (4 to 6 year) children took halting steps with much flailing about. More and more of the older (9 to 15 year)
children walked rapidly and smoothly. These results agree with those of
Olson (13) who has also noted that balancing reactions improve with age.

Thompson's (17) studies of extent of muscular involvement a n d studies of
how children learn to walk, skate, jump, throw, climb, bicycle, and w r i t e,
by McGraw (11), Halverson (8), Gutterridge (7), Buhler (2), S h i r l e y (14),
Gesell (5), Merry (12), Cron (3), and Strickland (16), indicate s i m i l a r i m-
provement with age.

Girls averaged definitely better than boys in walking the balance board in
age groups 4 to 8, but in the 8 to 15 age group, boys averaged better. Jenkins
(10) found that girls 5, 6 and 7 years of age surpassed boys i n t h e ability to
hop on one foot, a performance requiring "sense of balance". B u h l e r (2)
noted fewer superfluous movements among girls than among boys age 6 and 7.
However, Gesell (6) found that boys excel in throwing and running a t 5 to 7
years of age. After age 13 girls appear to decline somewhat in athletic ability and dynamic strength according to Stoddard and E s p e n s c h a d e (4), and
Ausubel (1).

The 13 to 15 year age girls, frequently more self conscious than other
groups, appeared hesitant to venture onto the balance board. At two of the
playgrounds where the balance board was put in a room and only one child at a
time admitted in to try walking it, the older girls averaged 2.5 while a t t w o
others where all the children attending the playground gathered a r o u n d, and
competition was keenest, the older girls averaged only 1.4.

In a recent study of the Lincoln Adaptation of the Oseretsky Test, Sloan (15)
found that males out-performed females in motor coordination f r o m a g e s 7
through 11 while females seemed to perform slightly better than males at age
levels 6 and 13. At ages 12 and 14 male and female scores were comparable.

We noted extreme individual differences in the performance of our subjects.
While most of the 4 to 6 year group scored "0", four of the 13 to 15 year olds
scored only one or two points. A glance at Table II will show that a p p r o x i-
mately 10 percent of the entire group was unable to score, while 7 p e r c e n t
made perfect scores. Several of the 11 to 15 year olds took halting steps like
a child from the 4 to 6 year group while several 7 and 8 year o l d s displayed
the same poise and smoothness as some children in the 11 to 15 age group.

While not fully explored in the present study, there was a suggestion t h a t
cultural factors had much to do with our subjects' performance on the balance
board. In his study, Sloan (15) pointed out that the motor skill of the e x a m-
iner may well be a variable in the performance of the subject. O n e w h o is
adept at a motor task may give the impression that it can be done easily. But
what caught our attention was the way our subjects approached the task, some

TABLE I

SHOWING DISTRIBUTION OF BALANCE BOARD SCORES
BY SEX AND AGE GROUPS

Age Groups	Boys' Scores							Ave.	Girls' Scores							Ave.	N	Totals Ave.
	0	1	2	3	4	5	6		0	1	2	3	4	5	6			
13-15	3	2	2	8	11	2	7	3.7	1	7	4	5	2	0	0	2.0	54	3.1
12-13	2	1	7	4	12	6	4	3.6	2	6	2	7	3	0	1	2.3	57	3.1
11-12	0	3	4	8	7	6	6	3.8	2	3	3	5	3	2	0	2.5	52	3.3
10-11	3	9	6	5	7	8	3	3.0	2	5	4	6	0	4	0	2.4	62	2.8
9-10	2	8	7	7	5	4	3	2.8	5	4	7	7	4	1	0	2.1	64	2.5
8- 9	7	11	8	9	11	2	2	2.5	7	6	6	5	4	2	0	2.0	80	2.3
7- 8	12	10	9	7	0	4	0	1.6	5	3	3	3	3	2	0	2.1	61	1.8
6- 7	17	11	7	1	0	1	0	0.9	3	2	3	2	1	0	0	1.6	48	1.1
4- 6	10	1	0	0	0	0	0	0.1	9	1	2	0	0	0	0	0.5	23	0.3

No. children tested, 501; no. boys, 322; no. girls, 179.

Method of scoring: Each child was given three trials at walking the balance board.
A miss, stepping off the board, scored 0.
Walking the length of the board before stepping off scored 1.
Walking length of board, turning and walking back ("round trip") scored 2.
A perfect score was 6.

TABLE II

PERCENTAGE OF ENTIRE GROUP
EARNING A GIVEN SCORE

				SCORES					
	0	1	2	3	4	5	6		Totals
Boys	17	34	34	41	53	28	25		232
Girls	19	31	26	35	16	9	1		137
Total	36	65	60	76	69	37	26		369
Percent	10	17 1/2	16	21	18 1/2	10	7		100

49

with confidence and others with great caution. Heath (9) has even suggested a possible relationship between motor performance and social adjustments. Again, we noticed that some children wished to perform first and before an audience while others would hang back wanting to try it out alone.

It is such observations as these that impel us towards a repetition of our study under conditions of competition vs. non-competition, using the present results as a comparison base. The significant question is: What is the effect of the presence of others on such a simple task as we observed in this experiment? Do the norms commonly published take such factors into consideration? Indeed, can competition really be controlled in our strongly competitive culture? Further research should throw some light on such fundamental questions.

REFERENCES

1. Ausubel, D. P. Theory and Problems of Adolescent Development, New York: G. Stratton Co. , 1954.
2. Buhler, Charlotte. From Birth to Maturity, London: K. Paul, Trench, Trubner and Co. Ltd. , 1935, pp. 117-146.
3. Cron, Gerald W. Parent Teacher Association Safety Drive, Wichita, Kansas: Fairmount School, 1954, (unpublished manuscript).
4. Espenschade, Anna. "Development of Motor Coordination in Boys and Girls," Research Quarterly American Association for Health and Physical Education, XVIII, 1947, pp. 30-43.
5. Gesell, Arnold. Infancy and Human Growth, New York: MacMillan Co. , 1928, pp. 132-133.
6. Gesell, Arnold. The Child From Five to Ten, New York: Harper, 1946, pp. 224-233.
7. Gutteridge, M. V. "A Study of Motor Achievement of Young Children," Archives of Psychology, 1939, p. 244.
8. Halverson, H. M. "An Experimental Study of Prehension In Infants," Genetics of Psychology Monograph, X, 1931.
9. Heath, R. S. "Clinical Significance of Motor Defect With Military Implications," American Journal of Psychology, LVII, 1944, pp. 482-489.
10. Jenkins, L. M. Motor Achievement of Children Five to Seven, New York: Teachers College, Columbia University, 1930, pp. 50-52.
11. McGraw, M. B. Growth, A Study of Johnny and Jimmy, New York: D. Appleton, 1935, pp. 20-21, 190-191.
12. Merry, F. K. and R. V. First Two Decades of Life, New York: Harpers, 1950, pp. 143-144.
13. Olson, W. C. Child Development, New York: Heath and Co. , 1949.
14. Shirley, M. M. The First Two Years, Minneapolis: University of Minnesota Press, 1931.
15. Sloan, William. "The Lincoln-Oseretsky Motor Development Seals," Genetics of Psychology Monograph, LI, 1955, pp. 183-252.
16. Strickland, Ruth. Language Arts, New York: Heath and Co. , 1951, pp. 233-234.
17. Thompson, G. G. Child Psychology, Boston: Houghton, Mifflin Co. , 1952, pp. 239-287.

RELIABILITY OF PERCEPTUAL-MOTOR LATERALITY TASKS

ALLAN BERMAN

Summary.—Test-retest and item-analysis reliability studies were performed on a battery of perceptual-motor laterality tasks. It was found that 45 of 54 tasks were reliable and that the entire battery had a test-retest correlation of .84. It was suggested that intermodal tasks may be more appropriate than unimodal tasks for measuring perceptual-motor skills. Suggestions were made for future research, emphasizing the need for more intermodal tasks, as well as the need for further reliability studies with more diverse sample groups.

Despite the long history of interest and research in the areas of laterality and cerebral dominance, there still remain serious questions about the reliability and validity of laterality measures. Although there have been a few widely disseminated standardized laterality measures, such as the one developed by Harris (1955, 1957); they can generally be criticized for lack of reliability or validity information. In addition, Berman (1971) has pointed out the need for developing laterality measures which discriminate continuously through the laterality range rather than simply dichotomize laterality as left or right.

Research continues to support the relationship between laterality or other perceptual-motor functions and various indicators of intellectual or academic ability (Miller, 1971; Berman, 1971; Groden, 1969; Levy, 1969). The tendency also still exists to assume that observed perceptual-motor laterality is related to the physiological concept of cerebral dominance, and the findings of Levy (1969) and others may be interpreted in such a manner. Although there is considerable speculation, there is as yet no demonstrated way of confirming the relationship between observed laterality and the concept of cerebral dominance.

This research is an effort to provide reliability information on a battery of laterality measures first introduced by Berman (1971), and called the Index of Cerebral Dominance. It is now felt that it would be more accurate and less presumptive to use the name Index of Perceptual-motor Laterality to refer to this battery.

Subjects

Ss were 98 children, ages 8 through 13 yr., ranging in intelligence from 45 to 140 IQ, matched individually for intelligence and age with the original sample (Berman, 1971).

Measurements

The Columbia Mental Maturity Scale, a short, reliable intelligence measure, was used. This test can be administered completely nonverbally and does not re-

PERCEPTUAL MOTOR SKILLS, 1973, Vol. 36, pp. 599-605.

quire a verbal response. The scale has high correlations with other standard IQ tests.

Tasks used to measure laterality are listed below. They include some originals as well as some which were obtained from those used and found to be reliable by Luria (1966), Coleman and Deutsch (1964), Delacato (1963), Greenberg (1960), Harris (1957, 1955), Lieben (1951), and Van Riper (1934). Tasks were randomized to determine order of administration. Ss were given the following instructions:

"I'm going to ask you to do some things. Listen carefully and make sure you do exactly as I say. If you don't understand something, or if you want me to repeat it, don't be afraid to ask."

(1) "Fold your hands like this." (Demonstration of folding with interlocking fingers. Dominant hand indicated by outermost thumb.)

(2, 3) "Draw a circle. . . . Now do it with the other hand . . . Now do it with both hands at the same time." (Record which hand was used first, and which circle was more accurately drawn.)

(4) "Let me see you hop on one leg." (Record which leg was used.)

(5, 6) "Hold this pencil in your hand right here (10 in. directly in front of S's nose). Now close one eye. Now open that eye and close the other. When did the pencil look like it was higher?" (E may repeat if necessary. Record which hand was used, and which eye was closed when pencil seemed higher.)

(7, 8) Administration of the Purdue Pegboard for right hand, left hand, and both hands together, using directions and standardized norms provided with that test. (Record which hand achieved better score separately, and which hand achieved better score when both were used together.)

(9, 10) "Put your ear against that wall and tell me if you hear anything. (Motion to wall to S's right.) Now put your ear against that wall and tell me if you hear anything." (Motion to wall to S's left. Record which ear was used each time.)

(11) "Stand up. Close your eyes and put your feet together. Now lift up your arms and hold them straight out in front of you." (Record which arm was higher.)

(12, 13) "See if you can throw this ball into the basket from here (10 feet away). Now try it with your other hand." (Record which hand was used first and which was more accurate.)

(14) "Fold your arms like this." (Demonstrate. Record which arm was uppermost.)

(15) "Step up on this chair. Now step down." (Record which foot was used to step down.)

(16) "Put your arms on the table with your hands together like this. Now push as hard as you can with both hands." (Record hand opposite direction of tilt.)

(17) "Can you write your name? Do the best you can." (While *S* wrote, *E* noticed from rear the direction of head tilt. Record opposite eye as dominant.)

(18, 19, 20) "I want to see how well you can kick. Stand here (10 ft. away) and see if you can kick the ball to me. (Ball placed 2 ft. to left of *S*.) Now try it again. (Ball placed directly in front of *S*.) Now once more." (Ball placed 2 ft. to right of *S*. Record foot used each time.)

(21, 22) "Let me see you cut this paper on that line with the scissors. Now try it with the other hand." (Record which hand was used first and which was more accurate. Two measurements.)

(23, 24) "Draw a square. Now do it with the other hand. Now do it with both hands at the same time." (Record which hand was used first and which drew the more accurate square.)

(25) "Kneel down on one knee." (Record which knee.)

(26, 27) "Put this paper in front of you so that you can see the 'X' clearly. Now take this (3½ in.) tube in one hand and look through it so you can see the 'X'. Now bring the tube up to one eye so that you can still see the 'X'." (Record which hand was used and which eye was used.)

(28, 29) "Walk over to the door. Stop facing the door. Now when you come back, walk backward." (Record foot used first walking forward and foot used first walking backward.)

(30, 31) "Aim this rifle and pretend you're going to shoot me." (Record which hand was used for trigger and which eye was used for sighting.)

(32, 33) "Put some beads on this string. Now do it with the other hand." (This was timed, using Stanford-Binet beads. Record which hand was used first and which hand strung more beads in one minute.)

(34, 35, 36) "Hold this pencil in your hand like this. Now place the pencil so it is even with the line on that wall. Now close one eye. Does the pencil move? Now close the other eye. Did the pencil move that time?" (Record which hand was used, which eye was closed first, and which eye caused movement of the pencil when closed.)

(37, 38) "Write your name. Now do it with the other hand. Now do it with both hands together." (Record which hand was used first, and which hand was better controlled.)

(39, 40) "Take this paper in one hand and hold it straight out so you can see that red mark on the wall through this hole in the paper. Now bring the paper up to your eye so you can still see the red mark." (Record hand and eye used.)

(41, 42, 43) (Stopwatch was placed on table 2 ft. to left of *S*.) "Put your ear down on this watch and listen to the ticking. (Watch was moved to a position directly in front of *S*.) Now listen once more. (Watch was moved to 2 ft. to right of *S*.) Now listen again." (Record which ear used each time.)

(44, 45) "Hold this (10 in.) tube up to your eye with one hand so you can see the red spot on the wall." (Record which hand was used and which eye was used.)

(46, 47, 48) "See if you can break this paper cup with your foot. (Cup placed 2 ft. to right of S.) Now break this one. (Cup placed directly in front of S.) Now this one." (Cup placed 2 ft. to left of S. Record which foot was used each time.)

(49, 50) "Let me show you how to wind this stopwatch. Now you do it for me. Now try it with the other hand." (Record which hand was used first and which was more efficient.)

(51) "Step up onto this chair." (S was placed directly in front of chair with feet together prior to directions. Record which foot was used to step up.)

(52, 53) "Hammer this nail into the board. Now try it with the other hand." (Record which hand was used first and which was more accurate.)

(54) (Boys) "Swing this bat for me." (Girls) "Show me how you sweep the floor with this broom." (Record which hand was used as power hand.)

Procedure

In all cases Ss were administered the Columbia Mental Maturity Scale first, to determine whether Ss would be appropriate for the sample and to help in matching. Ss were matched individually for IQ and age with the earlier sample (Berman, 1971). Immediately afterward the battery was administered in the order listed. The entire procedure required 35 to 50 min. per S. All Ss were tested individually, and the battery was run through twice per S.

RESULTS

A test-retest correlation of .84 was obtained for the first and second administrations of the battery for each S.

The test-retest correlation was not significantly different from that obtained for the original sample ($r = .86$, Berman, 1971). This apparently would strengthen the stability of the battery as a measure. In addition, an internal consistency item-analysis was performed using a biserial correlation coefficient (see Table 1). Of the 54 measurements, 9 were insignificantly related to total laterality scores: two hand measures, 3 foot measures, and 4 ear measures. All eye measures were significant.

The item-analysis suggests that 9 items should be omitted from the battery to increase internal consistency. Interestingly, 4 of these are ear tasks. There were only five ear tasks initially, suggesting the possibility that ear laterality may be inherently unreliable in affecting over-all laterality patterns. Groden's results, however, (1969) suggest that there are items which do consistently measure hand/ear laterality. This aspect is one that will have to be investigated further.

TABLE 1
RESULTS OF BISERIAL CORRELATION ITEM-ANALYSIS OF LATERALITY TASKS

Measurement Numbers	Biserial r	CR	p	Measurement Numbers	Biserial r	CR	p
Hand Tasks				Foot Tasks			
1	−.1137	.947	NS	4	.4368	2.921	<.01
2	.6668	3.405	<.01	15	.3325	2.383	<.05
3	.5100	2.810	<.01	18	.6693	2.824	<.01
5	.5945	3.215	<.01	19	.5225	3.172	<.01
7	.4710	2.525	<.05	20	.5163	3.326	<.01
8	.3614	2.152	<.05	25	.2406	1.723	NS
11	.4055	2.800	<.01	28	.2380	1.772	NS
12	.4710	2.524	<.05	29	.3976	2.757	<.01
13	.2882	1.982	<.05	46	.4793	2.789	<.01
14	.0207	.162	NS	47	.4946	2.938	<.01
16	.4051	2.788	<.01	48	.4372	2.912	<.01
21	.5510	2.882	<.01	51	.1207	.931	NS
22	.4727	2.727	<.01				
23	.5900	3.013	<.01	Eye Tasks			
24	.5424	2.797	<.01	6	.3809	2.660	<.01
26	.4572	2.857	<.01	17	.4699	2.819	<.01
30	.3702	2.438	<.05	27	.2897	2.002	<.05
32	.2832	1.963	<.05	31	.3539	2.454	<.05
33	.3948	2.612	<.01	35	.4628	3.089	<.01
34	.3874	2.207	<.05	36	.4259	2.909	<.01
37	.5948	2.847	<.01	40	.4427	2.955	<.01
38	.5157	2.624	<.01	45	.4091	2.762	<.01
39	.6298	3.251	<.01				
44	.3806	2.407	<.05	Ear Tasks			
49	.5102	2.628	<.01	9	.1163	.895	NS
50	.6043	3.255	< .01	10	−.0885	.678	NS
52	.5607	2.604	<.01	41	.2982	2.078	<.05
53	.6337	3.273	<.01	42	.0721	.554	NS
54	.3201	2.288	<.05	43	.1746	1.327	NS

It has also been suggested by Bruml (1972), Berman (1971), Groden (1969), and others that complex intermodal tasks (i.e., tasks involving eye and hand, or ear and hand, etc.) may be more relevant to perceptual-motor efficiency than unimodal tasks involving one part of the body only. All of the insignificant tasks were unimodal. Table 2 lists the number and types of intermodal tasks in the battery. Most of them are hand/eye coordination tasks, and a few are foot/eye tasks. Future research should develop and evaluate additional foot/eye tasks, and there is a need for development of hand/ear and other intermodal coordination tasks. Bruml (1972) has also pointed out the need for differentiating between unimanual tasks and bimanual tasks, as well as between tasks requiring skill or accuracy, and those requiring speed of performance. Ammons

TABLE 2

NUMBER AND TYPE OF INTERMODAL TASKS INCLUDED IN LATERALITY MEASURE

Number of Task	Type of Task	Number of Task	Type of Task
2,3	hand/eye	30,31	hand/eye
5,6	hand/eye	32,33	hand/eye
7,8	hand/eye	34,35,36	hand/eye
12,13	hand/eye	37,38	hand/eye
17	hand/eye	39,40	hand/eye
18,19,20	foot/eye	44,45	hand/eye
21,22	hand/eye	46,47,48	foot/eye
23,24	hand/eye	49,50	hand/eye
26,27	hand/eye	52,53	hand/eye

and Ammons (1970) have evidence which supports the necessity for developing norms and reliability data for a wider range of subject variables, as well as a need to study such variables as performance decrement and cross-lateral transfer.

The present study does not enter the controversy about the validity of the relationship between perceptual-motor laterality and intellectual skills. This question has been dealt with by many researchers, and there is considerable evidence to support such a relationship (Satz, Achenbach, & Fennell, 1967; Knox & Boone, 1970; Berman, 1971). Nevertheless, many studies are inconclusive and the total picture is still unclear. It is felt that one reason for this may be the lack of a widely accepted, reliable series of laterality measurements. The present research, while not yet definitive, is a step in that direction.

REFERENCES

AMMONS, R. B., & AMMONS, C. H. Decremental and related processes in skilled performance. In L. E. Smith (Ed.), *Psychology of motor learning, Proceedings of C.I.C. Symposium on Psychology of Motor Learning, University of Iowa, October 10-12, 1969.* Chicago: Athletic Institute, 1970. Pp. 205-238.

BERMAN, A. The problem of assessing cerebral dominance and its relationship to intelligence. *Cortex,* 1971, 7, 372-386.

BRUML, H. Age changes in preference and skill measures of handedness. *Perceptual and Motor Skills,* 1972, 34, 3-14.

COLEMAN, R., & DEUTSCH, C. P. Lateral dominance and right-left discrimination: a comparison of normal and retarded readers. *Perceptual and Motor Skills,* 1964, 19, 43-50.

DELACATO, M. *The diagnosis and treatment of speech and reading problems.* Springfield, Ill.: Thomas, 1963.

GREENBERG, G. Eye dominance and head tilt. *American Journal of Psychology,* 1960, 73, 149-151.

GRODEN, G. Lateral preferences in normal children. *Perceptual and Motor Skills,* 1969, 28, 213-214.

HARRIS, J. *The Harris Tests of Lateral Dominance.* New York: Psychological Corp., 1955.

HARRIS, J. Lateral dominance, directional confusion, and reading disability. *Journal of Psychology,* 1957, 44, 238-294.

KNOX, A. W., & BOONE, D. R. Auditory laterality and total handedness. *Cortex,* 1970, 6, 164-173.

LEVY, J. Possible basis for the evaluation of lateral specialization of the human brain. *Nature*, 1969, 224, 614-615.

LIEBEN, B. Analysis of the results of the Harris Tests of Lateral Dominance used as group tests. Unpublished Master's thesis, City College of New York, 1951.

LURIA, A. R. *Higher cortical functions in man.* New York: Basic Books, 1966.

MILLER, E. Handedness and the pattern of human ability. *British Journal of Psychology*, 1971, 62, 111-112.

SATZ, P., ACHENBACH, K., & FENNELL, E. Correlations between assessed manual laterality and predicted speech laterality in a normal population. *Neuropsychologia*, 1967, 5, 295-310.

VAN RIPER, C. A new test of laterality. *Journal of Experimental Psychology*, 1934, 18, 372-382.

PART II

LOCOMOTION

DELAYED EMERGENCE OF PRONE LOCOMOTION

DAVID A. FREEDMAN, M.D.[1] AND CAY CANNADY, A.B.

Delay in the emergence of crawling behavior was observed in a group of seven children. Each was followed from a state of total locomotor immobility to skilled creeping and crawling. Despite the remarkable (up to 1 year) retardation, the pattern of emergence of crawling was generally consistent with that described by McGraw for normally developing children. A notable exception was the tendency of delayed children to begin forward locomotion before they could raise their abdomens off the supporting surface. This finding, taken together with the fact that the most significant delay was found in two anatomically intact individuals who had suffered massive environmental deprivation, suggests that the emergence of typical patterns of prone progression is dependent on adequate very early somesthetic stimulation.

We have had the opportunity to study seven children who showed significant delay in the initiation of horizontal locomotion. In each case our observations embraced the period from total locomotor immobility to skillful crawling. McGraw's (13, 14) study of the emergence of patterns of locomotion in normal infants provided us with a set of norms against which it was possible to evaluate our data. We present our findings as a contribution to the ever present problem of the relative roles of endogenous and environmental factors in the evolution of behavior.

McGRAW'S FINDINGS

The emergence of patterns of prone progression is one of the items McGraw included in her investigation of the neuromuscular development of the human infant. On the basis of 1777 observations in a group of 82 infants, she was able to identify nine phases in the evolution of crawling and creeping (Figure 1). With the exception of

[1] Baylor Medical College, Houston, Texas, and New Orleans Psychoanalytic Institute, New Orleans, Louisiana.

This report is based on studies supported by National Institute of Health and Child Development Grant HD02763 and Grant 2-2971, General Research Funds, Baylor College of Medicine.

a few instances in which F and G were reversed, the phases emerged in an invariant sequence. She did note, however, that later phases tended to emerge during the period of their predecessors maximal activity, and only gradually to replace them. Figure 2, prepared from McGraw's data, shows the age range of her subjects at the time of the emergence of each phase. Particularly noteworthy from the standpoint of our observations is the evidence that reversal of phases F and G occurred in association with relative delay in the evolution of crawling.

METHOD AND CLINICAL MATERIAL

The subjects reported here were being followed in connection with a broader study of the effects of congenital and perinatal sensory deprivations on the process of ego formation. With rare exceptions, they were seen at monthly intervals in their homes. Both written and motion picture records were made of each session.

For the purpose of the present investigation, the records were reviewed and the age at which each of McGraw's phases was first observed was determined. Relevant clinical data are presented in the following vignettes. Table 1 summarizes the clinical diagnoses.

JOURNAL OF NERVOUS AND MENTAL DISEASES, 1971, Vol. 153, pp. 108-117.

60

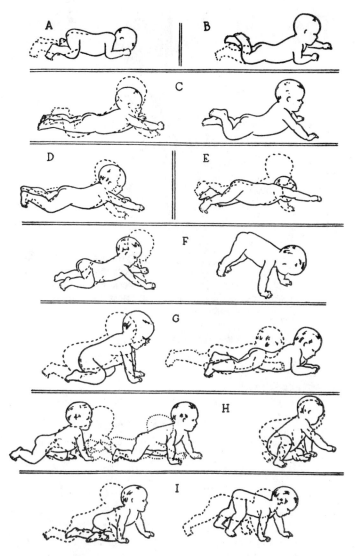

Fig. 1. Nine phases in the development of prone progression. (From McGraw, M. B., J. Genet. Psychol., Columbia University Press, *58*: 83–111, 1941.)

1. T. A. BLIND FROM BIRTH AS A RESULT OF OPHTHALMIA NEONATORUM

Pregnancy and delivery were described as uneventful. The youngest of a sibship of five, T. was fathered out of wedlock. Her mother, who had been deserted by her husband after the birth of the next older sibling, was depressed for some months following T.'s birth. Aside from the blindness, T.'s physical status was not remarkable. This child was followed from her 5th through her 30th month. Extended observations of other aspects of her development have been reported elsewhere (6).

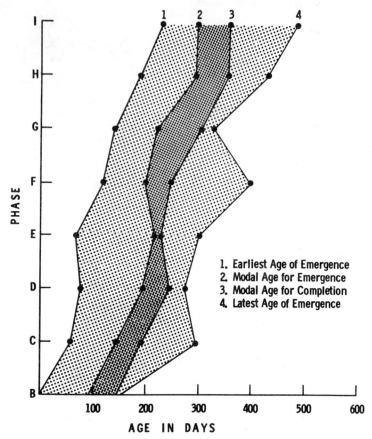

FIG. 2. Distribution of McGraw's 82 infants as to their manifestations of nine phases in the development of prone progression (prepared from McGraw's 1941 data).

2. J. R. ANOPHTHALMIA

Pregnancy and delivery were uneventful. Birth weight was 6 lb, 7 oz. J. is the younger of two brothers. The diagnosis was made at the time of the birth of this otherwise healthy youngster. From the available external evidence, mother appears to have responded to the fact of his blindness with the determination that he be treated like a "normal" child. Observations of his developmental progress were initiated when he was 10 weeks old and have continued at monthly intervals since then.

3. C. K. CONGENITAL RUBELLA COMPLICATED BY BILATERAL CATARACTS, PATENT DUCTUS ARTERIOSUS, SOME DEGREE OF DEAFNESS, AND POSSIBLE ENVIRONMENTAL DEPRIVATION

Aspects of this child's developmental progress have been reported elsewhere (7). Pregnancy and delivery were uneventful. The diagnosis of congenital rubella was made at birth. He weighed 5 lb, 4 oz. At 6 months the patent ductus was repaired, and 1 month later the cataracts were removed. Nonetheless, marked developmental delay has persisted. The complexities of the problem he presents are indicated by his inclusion in all three of our diagnostic categories (Table 1). The combination of chronic air hunger and blindness during his first 6 months seems to us to have served as a barrier to environmental stimulation so that despite considerable attention from his mother, he was in effect understimulated.

4. D. W. CONGENITAL RUBELLA COMPLICATED BY UNILATERAL CATARACT AND DEAFNESS

Because of fetal cardiac irregularities, delivery was by cesarean section. She weighed 5 lb, 6 oz at birth. Our observations began when she was 3 months old. Like many rubella babies, she expressed displeasure when held in the vertical position (3), but appeared calm and content when prone or supine. This response, which persisted until she was 8 months old, was interpreted by mother as rejection. Bilateral hearing loss on the order of 80 db has been established.

5. A. P. CONGENITAL RUBELLA, DEAFNESS, AND ENVIRONMENTAL DEPRIVATION

Birth weight was 5 lb, 8 oz, and delivery by midwife was uneventful. Mother was hospitalized with tuberculosis 1 week post partum, and A. was placed in foster care at 21 days. A persisting subcutaneous eruption and failure to thrive led to his being hospitalized when he was 9 months, 20 days. Developmental status at that time was reported to be compatible with that of a child of 2 to 3 months. A diagnosis of active rubella infection was made, and A. was kept in isolation until we observed him at 1 year, 2 months, 20 days. Examination revealed a friendly baby who showed much visual interest in his surroundings. He was unable to sit unsupported. Head lag was present when he was held supine. He would roll from side to side but could not turn over from either the prone or supine position. Bilateral hearing loss on the order of 80 db was demonstrated. He was placed in foster care at 1

year, 4 months, 17 days. Serological indices of rubella infection have persisted throughout the period of observation.

6. S. B. ENVIRONMENTAL DEPRIVATION

S. is fifth in a sibship of six. Mother was deserted by her husband during pregnancy with this child. Delivery was uncomplicated. Apgar index was 8 (1). Birth weight was 5 lb, 7 oz. From his 19th to his 58th day, the child was hospitalized for the treatment of multiple rat bites on his face. At 5 months, 18 days, he was again hospitalized with the diagnosis of failure to thrive and salmonella septicemia. We were consulted during his third admission for failure to thrive. He was 21 months old and weighed 11 lb, 8 oz. He was able to support himself on his forearms in a posture compatible with McGraw's phase C.

7. T. B. ENVIRONMENTAL DEPRIVATION

Younger half-brother of S. B. At time of delivery, mother was considered preeclamptic. Apgar index, however, was 9, and delivery was uneventful. Birth weight was 9 lb, 8 oz. A grade II to III basal systolic murmur was recorded, and there was some question of hypertonicity of the lower extremities. The child, however, progressed well during 7 days of post partal hospitalization. When he was hospitalized at 3 months with the diagnosis of enterocolitis and malnutrition, his weight was 7 lb, 14 oz; i.e., nearly 2 lb under his birth weight. During a hospital stay of 21 days, he gained 3 lb. Three months later (at the same time S. B. was referred), when T. was readmitted and referred to us, he weighed (at 7 months), 8 lb, 4 oz. He could raise his head when he was placed in the prone position. Head lag persisted, however, when he was held supine. At 1 year, 3 months, 28 days, he made no effort of locomotion, and showed no interest in reaching for or grasping available objects. Prone progression was first observed at 21 months. Progress thereafter was rapid until 23 months, when T. was found dead in his crib. Post mortem examination revealed bilateral bronchopneumonia. Aside from this and the unusually small size of the body (length, 29 inches; weight, 17 lb), the autopsy findings were within normal limits. There was no evidence of nutritional deficiency. The brain of this subject will be the subject of a separate report.

OBSERVATIONS

Our findings are summarized in Figures 3, 4, and 5. For clarity of presentation we have segregated the subjects according to the diagnoses in Table 1. As a consequence, the curve for C. K. is included in all three figures, and that for A. P. in those for the rubella children and the environmentally deprived (Figures 4 and 5). Despite their greater age, emergence of prone progression in our subjects, once it began, followed the pattern described by McGraw. The cephalocaudal sequence of emergence was as characteristic of these children as it was of her normally developing population.

Environmental deprivation appears to be more likely to yield significant delay in the emergence of prone progression than is either the somatic sequelae of congenital rubella, or the absence of visual input. As a group, the four environmentally deprived

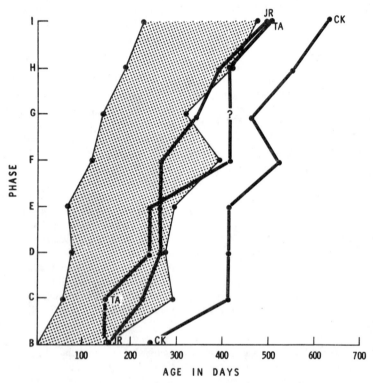

Age Range for Emergence of Phases in McGraw's 82 Infants (McGraw 1941)
—?— Indicates no observations were made of the Phase

FIG. 3. The first appearance of each phase of prone progression as manifested by congenitally blind children.

64

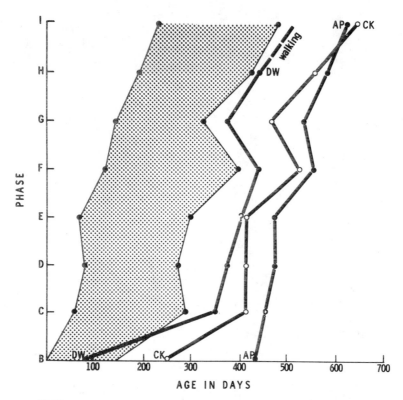

Fig. 4. The first appearance of each phase of prone progression as manifested by rubella children.

subjects were the most delayed in both the inception and evolution of horizontal locomotion. Within the environmentally deprived group, furthermore, it was the two children who were born with least evidence of congenital somatic problems who were most retarded.

The ability to carry the body forward, i.e., prone locomotion of any form, was designated by McGraw as phase G. With rare exceptions she found that this appeared after the child was able to maintain its abdomen above the supporting surface (phase F). Although McGraw was not explicit in this regard, we infer from her data (curve 3 in Figure 2; shaded areas in Figures 3, 4,

and 5) that the phase reversal occurred most frequently in those of her subjects who were relatively delayed in developing crawling behavior. All four of the children we include in our environmentally deprived group showed this reversal (Figure 5). All four children passed through a relatively long period typical of McGraw's phases D and E. Three of the four remained at this level and were unable to lift their abdomens from the supporting surface for 82 to 111 days. Characteristically during this period, when an object was placed within arm's length of the child, he could retrieve it without difficulty. If, however, the object was placed beyond the subject's grasp, even

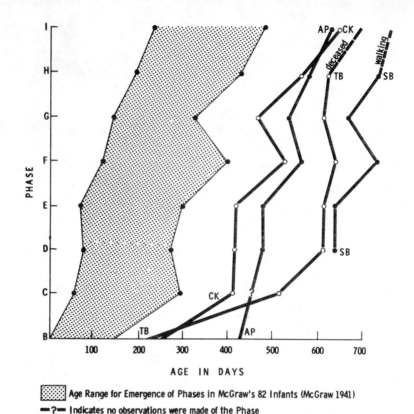

Fig. 5. The first appearance of each phase of prone progression as manifested by environmentally deprived children.

TABLE 1
Classification of Subjects according to Diagnostic Categories

Subject	Congenital Blindness	Congenital Rubella	Environmental Deprivation
T. A.	x		
J. R.	x		
C. K.	x	x	?
D. W.		x	
A. P.		x	x
S. B.			x
T. B.			x

if he could brush it with his fingertips, he was helpless. Although he would reach and strain and at times his legs would kick, there was no semblance of forward movement. Progression, when it ultimately began, was slow and painful. To the observer with military experience, the youngster appeared to be caricaturing a soldier moving forward under fire. The ventral surface of the body was maintained in close proximity to the floor, and the propulsive force was provided by the arms and shoulders. At first the lower extremities were simply dragged along. Over a period of 30 to 50 days, the child gradually acquired the ability to flex his knees, and finally he raised his abdomen from the floor.

DISCUSSION

Data from a variety of sources (2, 9) have established that within the population of "normal babies," a considerable range of

66

responsivity is found from birth onward. At any given age, mothering which may be entirely adequate for one infant's needs may be inadequate for another's. In addition to the available environment, the infant's capacity to respond to proffered stimulation serves to determine what from the world around it he will ultimately incorporate. Escalona (4) has designated the resultant of the interaction of the child's organismic potentialities and the environment, "patterns of concrete experience." She points out that essentially equivalent patterns of concrete experience may be the result of highly varying combinations of endogenous (organismic) factors and environmental input.

She conceives of development as a process of continuing modifications of the organism. These are derived from the interaction of new patterns of concrete experience, the residual effects of prior experience, and the results of endogenous, gene-determined maturational processes. In Piaget's (15) terms, maturation of the central nervous system per se simply opens up the possibility for new responses and functional developments; it does not result in the actualization of any given response unless appropriate environmental circumstances are available.

The study of "average expectable" infants in an "average expectable" environment, to use Hartmann's (11) phrase, tends to gloss over these considerations and make possible the assumption that at least for the early years (10), the development of the child amounts to little more than an unfolding of innate abilities. Such a point of view has been widely supported in the past (e.g., Tilney and Cassamajor [17]; Tilney and Kubie [18]). McGraw (14), for example, has stated, "... as soon as the maturation of all neural centers involved is complete, the baby tends to employ a more conventional mode of creeping" (p. 58). Our observations are not congruent with such a conclusion. It would appear that in the absence of time-appropriate envirnomental input,

relevant organismic modifications are either significantly delayed or fail entirely to emerge, *even if neural maturation is proceeding on schedule.*

It is particularly impressive that the most significant developmental disturbances occurred in those of our youngsters whose patterns of concrete experience were least limited by endogenous factors. Environmental deprivation predicated on maternal neglect was associated with the most dramatic delays in the emergence and maturation of patterns of horizontal locomotion. Even in the group of four youngsters whom we consider environmentally deprived, it was the one with the most significant congenital tissue pathology but who received the most maternal attention who was least delayed in the development of crawling.

Congenital blindness in otherwise intact youngsters, resulted in a relatively minor delay in development of prone locomotion. Despite the absence of a visual stimulus, emergences of the various phases described by McGraw were either within the range of those of her 82 normal subjects or only slightly beyond it. The one blind baby in whom we were able to record all the phases, initiated prone progression at 11½ months. It has already been established (5, 7), that in both blind and sighted children, searching behavior in response to auditory stimuli also emerges at approximately this age. We cite this coincidence because of the implication that when the otherwise normally developing blind child is able to use hearing cues to indicate the existence of something "out there," auditory stimuli may interact with the organismic state to yield a pattern of concrete experience equivalent to that which we ordinarily associate with visual input. The child then is able to respond with appropriate search and/or locomotor behavior.

On the other hand the environmentally deprived children with entirely adequate vision failed to initiate locomotor efforts until they were well into their 2nd year of life.

Such a dramatic delay, especially in subjects without evidence of significant congenital motor or sensory deficit cannot, we propose, be accounted for on the basis of failure of endogenous maturational processes. Neither, we feel, can it be adequately explained as a lack of interest in external objects. Among the more poignant observations we have made is the picture of such a child eagerly inspecting a bottle of milk barely beyond his reach. For periods of as much as 100 days, such an object might as well have been at the other end of the world. The child strains and reaches, but he is incapable of organizing his movements so as to produce forward motion. His head bobs up and down and his legs kick, but the movements have a random unintegrated quality. A similar lag has been described by Provence and Lipton (16) in infants confined to institutions. Although locomotion has preceded getting up on hands and knees, cephalocaudal progression in the evolution of crawling consistent with McGraw's description has occurred. The ages of our subjects, however, seem to preclude her assumption that this progression is a result of the process of neural maturation per se. As an alternative (one to which McGraw seems to be alluding in the introduction to the reprint of her monograph (14) page xvi), we propose that the delayed emergence and organization of crawling is related to a disturbance in the process of the organization of the anatomic substrata of body image. In this regard we cite the work of Held and Bauer (12). Their studies would seem to confirm that maturation of the nervous system per se does not lead to effective use of a given innervated part. They placed newborn, anatomically intact, primates in an apparatus which effectively deprived them of visual contact with their upper extremities. At 35 days, when the animal was allowed visual contact with one hand, visually guided reaching was poorly executed and only gradually improved. There was, furthermore, little concomitant improvement of the response in the opposite hand until it too had undergone a period of practice under the guidance of vision.

We interpret the reversal of phases F and G in our subjects as well as the children's behavior, prior to the inception of forward progression, as further evidence of failure to develop relevant patterns of brain organization in the absence of appropriate environmental stimulation. To use McGraw's phrase, "that strange thing called motivation" (13, page 93) to move toward an object usually becomes manifest after the child has acquired awareness of and some degree of control over his caudal parts. In our subjects, however, it appears to have been the case that the process of attempting prone locomotion provided the sensory input which in turn made the youngster aware of the existence of his lower extremities. The urge to move, in effect, preceded the development of the necessary equipment.

We feel the intermediate position occupied by the rubella babies (Figure 3) supports this assumption. They were more delayed than the congenitally blind, but less so than the purely environmentally deprived. Both D. W. and C. K., like many rubella babies (3), became irritable when they were held by their mothers. For C. K. this was, of course, complicated by the other problems we have enumerated. D. W., however, was sighted from birth and in no physical distress. Nonetheless, because she became irritable when she was held, she was rarely handled and fondled. We have no data for A. P. before his hospitalization at 9 months. Subsequently, however, we know that he was considered contagious and kept in isolation for some 5 months.

During this period he received excellent hygienic care. Play and handling, however, was available only to the extent that some member of the nursing staff with a few moments to spare might choose to spend them with him. Despite the absence of other evidence of somatic disease and excellent developmental progress once he entered foster care, he was more delayed in developing prone progression than either D. W. or C. K.

SUMMARY

Seven children characterized by delayed development of prone progression were followed from states of locomotor immobility to active crawling. Despite their advanced ages, the emergence of locomotor patterns in these subjects followed a course similar to that described by McGraw in 82 normally developing infants. The most striking delays in the emergence of patterns of crawling occurred in youngsters who showed no evidence of congenital somatic disease but had suffered severe environmental deprivation. The findings are interpreted to indicate that in the absence of age-appropriate environmental stimulation, neural maturation per se will not yield anticipated behavioral manifestations.

REFERENCES

1. Apgar, V. and James, L. S. Further observations on the newborn scoring system. Amer. J. Dis. Child., *104*: 419–428, 1962.
2. Bergman, P. and Escalona, S. K. Unusual sensitivities in very young children. In *Psychoanalytic Study of the Child,* vol. 3 and 4, pp. 333–352. International Universities Press, New York, 1949.
3. Desmond, M. M., Wilson, G. S., Verniaud, W. M., Melnick, J. L. and Rawls, W. E. The early growth and development of infants with congenital rubella. In Mordue, J. G., ed. *Advances in Teratology,* vol. 4, pp. 43–52. Logos Press, London. In press.
4. Escalona, S. K. Some determinants of individual differences. Trans. N. Y. Acad. Sci., *27*: 802–816, 1965.
5. Fraiberg, S. Parallel and divergent patterns in blind and sighted infants. In *The Psycho-*
analytic Study of the Child, vol. 23, pp. 264–300. International Universities Press, New York, 1968.
6. Fraiberg, S. and Freedman, D. A. Studies in the ego development of congenitally blind infants. In *The Psychoanalytic Study of the Child,* vol. 19, pp. 113–169. International Universities Press, New York, 1964.
7. Freedman, D. A., Fox-Kolenda, B. J. and Brown, S. L. A multihandicapped rubella baby; The first eighteen months. J. Amer. Acad. Child Psychiat., *9:* 298–317, 1970.
8. Freedman, D. A., Fox-Kolenda, B. J., Margileth, D. and Miller, D. H. The development of the use of sound as a guide to affective and cognitive behavior—A two phase process. Child Develop., *40:* 1099–1105, 1969.
9. Fries, M. E. and Woolf, P. J. Some hypotheses on the role of congenital activity type in personality development. In *Psychoanalytic Study of the Child,* vol. 8, pp. 448–469. International Universities Press, New York, 1953.
10. Gesell, A. and Armatruda, S. *Developmental Diagnosis,* 2nd ed. Hoeber, New York, 1960.
11. HARTMANN, H. *Ego Psychology and the Problem of Adaptation.* International Universities Press, New York, 1952.
12. Held, R. and Bauer, J. A. Visually guided reaching in monkeys after restricted rearing. Science, *155:* 718–720, 1967.
13. McGraw, M. B. Development of neuro-muscular mechanisms as reflected in the crawling and creeping behavior of the human infant. J. Genet. Psychol., *58:* 83–111, 1941.
14. McGraw, M. B. *The Neuro-Muscular Maturation of the Human Infant, 1945.* Reprint edition, Hafner, New York, 1963–1966.
15. Piaget, J. Problems of genetic psychology, (1956). Reprinted as Chapter 5 in Tenzer, Z., translator, *Six Psychological Studies,* pp. 116–131. Random House, New York, 1967.
16. Provence, S. and Lipton, R. C. *Infants in Institutions.* International Universities Press, New York, 1962.
17. Tilney, F. and Cassamajor, L. Myelinogeny as applied to the study of behavior. Arch. Neurol. (Chicago), *12:* 1–66, 1924.
18. Tilney, F. and Kubie, L. S. Behavior in its relation to the development of the brain. Bull. N. Y. Neurol. Inst., *1:* 229–311, 1931.

Effect of Rhythmic Accompaniment Upon Learning of Fundamental Motor Skills[1]

Gladys Lang Beisman

This study investigated the effect of rhythmic accompaniment upon the learning of the fundamental motor skills of throwing, catching, climbing, balancing, jumping, leaping, dodging, bouncing, and striking. Boys and girls (N = 607) in grades 1-6 were the subjects. Pre- and post-tests which were both qualitative and quantitative were administered. The period of treatment was 10 weeks. Analysis of the data supported the conclusion that rhythmic accompaniment, employed as a teaching technique for both boys and girls, can be expected to produce more improvement in performance during the development of fundamental motor skills at the elementary grade level than can teaching and practice without rhythmic accompaniment.

THE USE OF RHYTHMIC ACCOMPANIMENT in teaching appears to have desirable results. In the area of dance and rhythms music is essential and is allegedly conducive to equal or better accomplishment. A more pleasant atmosphere prevails when musical accompaniment becomes a part of the action. The implications this held for the development of fundamental motor skills for children led to this investigation.

Purpose

The purpose of this study was two-fold: (a) to test the effect of rhythmic accompaniment during instruction upon the style and performance of selected fundamental motor skills at each grade level, 1–6 and (b) to study sex differences in performance before and after the two treatments, and the differential effects of the treatments on the sex groups.

The skills selected for study were throwing, catching, climbing, and balancing for grades 1–3; jumping and leaping for each of the six grades; and dodging, bouncing, and striking for grades 4–6.

[1] This research study was an integral part of a doctoral study completed at the State University of New York at Buffalo, May, 1964. Acknowledgment is extended to Carlton R. Meyers.

RESEARCH QUARTERLY, 1967, Vol. 38, pp. 172-176.

Review of Literature

A great deal of research has been conducted in the areas of music and physical education which have bearing on rhythmic perception and performance, and fundamental motor skills. Efforts to relate the two disciplines have been fruitful in very limited areas and studies. General conclusions cannot be drawn from the evidence available. More research is needed in both areas with a greater understanding from a physiological, psychological, and musicological standpoint.

Dillon (1) conducted an experimental study as a means of measuring the value of music as an aid in teaching swimming. This value was determined by improvement in the speed and form of the crawl stroke and the breast stroke. The study was conducted over a period of three years and involved 240 college females of intermediate swimming ability. Dillon concluded that the swimmers who were taught with music improved more in swimming speed and in form than did the swimmers who were taught without music. It should be pointed out that swimmers of a different level of ability might or might not profit from the use of music, and that age and sex could influence the study. Further research seemed to be indicated.

Nelson (2) investigated the effect of selected rhythms and sound intensity on human performance as measured by the bicycle ergometer. No significant differences were found among any sets of conditions which varied music, pure tones, and music intensity. However, Nelson concluded that the results could conceivably be different when used in conjunction with the presence of other people and athletic competition.

Methodology

Sample. Boys and girls (N = 607) grades 1–6 from Durand-Eastman School, East Irondequoit, New York, were the subjects for the study conducted from January to June, 1963. There were four sections of grades 1, 2, 4, 5, and 6, and five sections of grade 3. Each section was heterogeneous with respect to academic potential, and each section had the same number of high, average, and low achievers. This was the established grouping policy for the school and was not altered for purposes of this study.

Two sections from each grade level were designated as the experimental group, and the remaining sections were used as the control group. Physical fitness and rhythmic aptitude information was used informally (visual comparison of data) in assigning groups to the treatment. An effort was made to avoid serious imbalance of the experimental and control groups on these variables. Another consideration was that the sequence of classes in the daily schedule did not entail a succession of either the control or the experimental groups. Each grade level met at the same time of day and all sections were taught by one teacher. The experimental and control groups were both given the same skills practice with identical number of repetitions. Every effort was made to have the rhythmic accompaniment as the single variable in the study.

Description of the tests. The fundamental skills employed in the study were evaluated before and after the treatment period on the basis of performance of a quantitative nature (how far, how fast, how often) and on the basis of rating of performance of a qualitative nature (how well, form, style). Two experienced judges performed the ratings. These judges saw the children only during the pre-tests and post-tests and did not know which groups had the rhythmic accompaniment.

The tests used for the specific skills were as follows: jumping, measured by the vertical jump; leaping, measured by the distance covered in four successive leaps; throwing, measured by an overhead accuracy test; catching, measured by the number of successful wall passes in 30 sec.; climbing, measured by the time required to ascend and descend a 15-foot ladder; balancing, measured by success in walking a balance board; dodging, measured by the time required to zigzag in and out of 12 swinging ropes; bouncing, measured by the time required to dribble a basketball in zigzag fashion around four benches; and striking, measured by the number of successful volleys completed in 30 sec. The ratings of the skills were made on a five-point scale employing a specific check list for each event and each participant. Each point on the rating scale, from 1 (poor) to 5 (superior), was stipulated in terms of performance; for example, for throwing, a rating of 1 was four or more misses, whereas 5 was without error. Ratings of the two judges were totaled for the final score. While no specific analysis was made, it was observed that agreement of judges appeared very close.

Statistical design. Pretests and post-tests were administered. Following the post-tests, the data for each test were analyzed separately at each grade level. The statistical design employed was a two-factor sex-by-treatment analysis of covariance using the pretest scores as the covariate. The data were processed on an IBM 1620 computer, and 66 analyses were performed.

The experimental variable was the rhythmic accompaniment. Other treatment variables were made as similar as possible through controlled practice time and number of repetitions, e.g., each lesson employing rhythmic accompaniment was analyzed as to the number of times the skill was to be repeated, and instructions were given to the control group to perform the action the same number of times. The rhythmic accompaniment was provided through the media of records, piano, tape recorder, dance drum, clapping, and singing. Records were employed a good deal of the time because it was felt that there would be greater application of the findings as a teaching technique in the event the rhythmic accompaniment proved significant. The treatment involved 10 weeks of practice on the selected skills. Not less than 10 nor more than 20 min. were spent during each of the two class sessions per week.

Results and Discussion

In 57 of the 66 analyses involved in the treatment (see Table 1), the experimental groups manifested significant improvement as contrasted to the control groups. In the remaining 9 analyses, although a significant difference was not indicated, improvement did occur in the desired direction. It must be noted, however, that of the 57 analyses that were significant an interaction that was also significant appeared in seven of the ratings and one of the

	Sex Grade						Treatment Grade						Interaction Grade					
	1	2	3	4	5	6	1	2	3	4	5	6	1	2	3	4	5	6
Throwing	B	O	BB				O	O	EE				O	O	O			
	B	BB	B				EE	EE	EE				O	O	*			
Catching	O	O	O				EE	EE	EE				O	O	O			
	O	O	B				EE	EE	EE				O	O	O			
Climbing	O	B	O				O	EE	EE				O	O	O			
	O	O	O				EE	O	O				O	O	O			
Balancing	GG	O	O				E	EE	EE				O	O	O			
	O	O	B				EE	EE	EE				O	O	O			
Jumping	O	O	O	O	O	O	EE	EE	EE	EE	EE	EE	O	O	O	O	O	O
	O	O	O	O	O	G	EE	EE	EE	EE	EE	EE	O	O	O	O	**	**
Leaping	O	O	O	O	O	O	EE	E	EE	EE	EE	E	O	O	O	O	O	*
	O	O	O	O	O	GG	EE	E	EE	EE	O	EE	O	O	O	O	**	O
Dodging			G	BB	O				EE	O	EE					O	O	O
			O	O	GG				EE	EE	O					O	*	*
Bouncing			B	O	O				EE	EE	EE					O	O	O
			BB	O	B				EE	EE	E					O	*	*
Striking			O	G	O				O	EE	EE					O	O	O
			B	O	O				EE	EE	EE					O	O	*

Underlining indicates rating score
Nonunderlining indicates performance score
O = No significant difference
B = Boys are significantly better (p < .05) than girls
BB = Boys are significantly better (p < .01) than girls
G = Girls are significantly better (p < .05) than boys
GG = Girls are significantly better (p < .01) than boys
E = Experimental group is significantly better (p < .05) than the control group
EE = Experimental group is significantly better (p < .01) than the control group
* = Interaction significant (p < .05)
** = Interaction significant (p < .01)

performance tasks. These interactions that were manifested between the two effects took place at the grades 5 and 6 level. It should be noted, however, that in these seven instances unusual motivating influences occurred with the control group of boys which were beyond the control of the investigator.

As shown in Table 1, little difference was noted between the performance of the boys and girls in the selected tasks. An exception was the throwing skill in which the boys, in five of the six analyses, were significantly superior to the girls. In the bouncing task the boys, at some levels, also demonstrated significant superiority over the girls in the performance of the skill. Significant differences between the performance of the boys and girls on some of the tests at some grade levels were found, but they permit no general statement. For example, in the skill of catching, third grade boys were significantly better (p < .05) in the rating than were the girls but there was no significant difference in the five other catching tests. Examination of Table 1 will reveal some other significant differences in test results between performance and rating scores of boys and girls. This examination will also support the general statement that there is little skill difference between boys and girls, with the exception of the throwing and bouncing tasks.

It was noted by visitors and classroom teachers during the course of the study that the groups being taught through the media of rhythmic accompaniments appeared to enjoy the activities more than did the control groups.

Conclusions

On the basis of an analysis of the findings of this investigation as presented herein, the following conclusion was drawn: Rhythmic accompaniment, employed as a teaching technique can be expected to produce more improvement in performance during the development of fundamental motor skills at the elementary grade level than can teaching and practice without rhythmic accompaniment.

On the basis of the complete findings of the original study, it was also concluded that:

1. A steady increase in the performance and ratings of the children can be anticipated across grade levels.

2. It would appear that the same methods can be employed for boys and girls during the teaching of the selected skills. All grades and both sexes improved as a result of the treatment, although the degree of improvement varied in some of the tasks and in some of the grades.

3. In throwing and bouncing tasks, boys can be expected to make greater gains than the girls at some levels. In the manner of performance of certain skills, upper grade girls can be expected to gain more than the boys under the treatment employing rhythmic accompaniment.

4. The rhythmic accompaniment can be expected to produce a relaxed and enjoyable atmosphere during the treatment.

The review of the literature of previous investigations, reported in the original study, did not show any particular method of teaching to be superior to any other. The expressed need was for more research related to specific skills and activities of the various grade levels. The evidence gathered in this study provides a definitive answer to the question of whether rhythmic accompaniment will result in better criterion performance of fundamental skills for grades 1-6 than will similar practice without rhythmic accompaniment.

References

1. DILLON, EVELYN K. A study of the use of music as an aid in teaching swimming. *Res. Quart.* 23:1-8, 1952.
2. NELSON, DALE O. Effect of selected rhythms and sound intensity on human performance as measured by the bicycle ergometer. *Res. Quart.* 34:484-88, 1963.

PART III

MANIPULATION

Observations on the Development of Visually-Directed Reaching

Burton L. White,* Peter Castle,[2]
and Richard Held

Brandeis University[3]

This paper reports the results of a normative study of the development of visually-directed prehension during the first six months of life. Thirty-four normal infants born and reared under relatively uniform conditions in a state hospital were studied. The technique combined detailed longitudinal observations with a standardized testing procedure designed to elicit visual-motor responses including prehension. A sequence of development is described, categorized into eight stages of two weeks each. A number of separate and distinct visual-motor and tactual motor behaviors were found to contribute to this sequence, culminating in the development of visually-directed reaching just prior to 5 months of age.

The prehensory abilities of man and other primates have long been regarded as one of the most significant evolutionary developments peculiar to this vertebrate group (2, 17). In man, the development of prehension is linked phylogenetically with the assumption of erect posture (thus freeing the forelimbs from the service of locomotion), the highly refined development of binocular vision, and the possession of an opposable thumb, among other specializations. One important accompaniment of the development of prehension is man's unique capacity to make and utilize tools. Considering the acknowledged importance of these developments in phylogeny, it is surprising how little is presently known about the ontogeny of prehension in

* Psychology Section, Department of Economics and Social Science, Massachusetts Institute of Technology, Cambridge 39, Massachusetts.

[1] This work was supported by Grant M-3657 from the National Institute of Mental Health, U. S. Public Health Service, and Grant 61-234 from the Foundation's Fund for Research in Psychiatry.

[2] Mr. Castle held a predoctoral fellowship from the National Institute of Mental Health while performing this research.

[3] The research was conducted at the Tewksbury Hospital, Tewksbury, Massachusetts. We are very grateful for the consideration and aid given by Dr. Lois Crowell and Head Nurses Helen Efstathiou and Frances Craig, among others.

CHILD DEVELOPMENT, 1964, Vol. 35, pp. 349-364.

man. The research to be presented here is focused on the behavioral ontogenesis of this vital function in the human infant during the first six months of life.

The detailed analysis of the development of a sensorimotor function such as prehension inevitably raises a classic theoretical problem. The human infant is born with a diversified reflex repertoire, and neuromuscular growth is rapid and complex. In addition, however, he begins immediately to interact with his postnatal environment. Thus we fact the complex task of distinguishing, to the extent that is possible, between those contributions made to this development by maturation or autogenous neurological growth and those which are critically dependent upon experience or some kind of informative contact with the environment. Previous work in the area of prehension has been variously oriented in regard to these polar alternatives, and it is important to note that the positions taken with regard to this theoretical problem have resulted in the gathering of selected kinds of data: namely, those kinds deemed relevant by each particular investigator to the support of his point of view on the development of prehension. Our own point of view is focused primarily around the role that certain kinds of experience have been shown to play in the growth and maintenance of sensorimotor coordinations (11). Consequently, we have focused our attention on gathering detailed longitudinal data of a kind that would aid us in eventually testing specific hypotheses about the contributions of such experience to the development of prehension.

Halverson (7) studied the reaching performance of infants, beginning only after the onset of what we have come to consider a rather advanced stage in the development of prehension (16 weeks). Gesell (5) used the response to single presentations of a dangling ring and a rattle as items in his developmental testing procedures. These tests were designed to be used with subjects as young as 4 weeks of age, but prehension was of only peripheral concern to Gesell. Both of these workers subscribed to the theoretical position, championed by Gesell, that most if not all of early growth, including the development of prehension, is almost exclusively a function of progressive neuromuscular maturation: an "unfolding" process. This view undoubtedly contributed to their neglect of the possible significance of the role of input from the sensory environment and to their stress on normative level of performance per se, rather than the relation between a level of performance and its behavioral antecedents.

Piaget (20) made a number of original observations on the development of prehension, including the earliest stages of the process, which are prior to 3 months of age. His data are somewhat limited since his subject group consisted only of his own three children. And, as with Gesell, Piaget's interest in prehension was peripheral to another concern, namely, the sensorimotor origins of intelligence. Piaget's theoretical approach differs considerably from that of Gesell, being concerned primarily with the cognitive aspects of development. His work is focused on the adaptive growth of intelligence or the capacity of the child to structure internally the results of his own actions. As a result, he has formulated a theoretical point of view that centers around the interaction of the child with his environment, an approach similar to our own. This interaction is seen by Piaget as giving rise to mental structures (schemas) which in turn alter the way in which the child will both perceive and respond to the environment subsequently. This point of view avoids the oversimplified dichotomy of maturation versus learning by conceptualizing development as an interaction process. Without the aliment provided by the environment schemas cannot develop, while without the existence of schemas the environment cannot be structured and thus come to "exist" for the child.

Some primitive sensorimotor schemas are, of course, present at birth, the grasp reflex and visual-motor pursuit being two that are particularly relevant to prehension. Both Gesell and Piaget describe the observable development of the subsequent coordination between vision and directed arm and hand movements, part of which is clearly dependent on some kind of practice or experience. Gesell, however, contented himself with a vague acknowledgment of the probable role of experience in development, whereas Piaget attempted to determine in a loose but experimental fashion the role of specific kinds of experiences and structured his theorizing explicitly around the details of the interaction process.

Piaget takes the position that informative contact with the environment plays an important role in the development of spatial coordination and, in particular, prehension. The work of Held and his collaborators (11, 13, 14, 15, 16) on the development and maintenance of plastic sensorimotor systems in higher mammals, including human adults, has led to a similar point of view. These laboratory studies have addressed themselves to the question of which specific kinds of contact with the environment are required for the maintenance and development of accurate sensorimotor abilities such as hand-eye coordination. This work constitutes a more rigorous experimental approach to some of the same kinds of problems that Piaget has dealt with on the basis of his extensive observations and seems likely to be relevant to the ontogeny of prehension in particular.

It was with this general framework in mind that we undertook the study of prehension. In studies of animal development (21, 22) the technique of selective deprivation of environmental contact has been successfully used to factor out critical determinants. Since human infants obviously cannot be deliberately deprived, other experimental strategies must be employed. One approach would be to enrich in selective fashion the environment of a relatively deprived group of infants, such as might be found in an institutional setting. The rate of development of such a group could then be compared with that of a similar group not receiving such enrichment. Under such conditions the differences might well be small and consequently the techniques of observation and measurement should be as precise and as sensitive as possible to detect systematic differences. Consequently, our first task was to determine in detail the normal sequence of behaviors relevant to prehension spanning the first six months of life. At the end of this time, visually-directed prehension is well developed. This preliminary information would enable us to devise sensitive and accurate scales for the measurement of prehension. We could then proceed with an examination of the role of contact with the environment in the development of this capacity. In addition, we felt that a detailed normative study of prehension was an important goal in its own right and one that would help fill an important gap in the study of human growth. It should be noted, however, that the results of this study can only be considered normative for subject groups such as ours.

METHOD

Subjects

Our subjects were 34 infants born and reared in an institution because of inadequate family conditions. These infants were selected from a larger group after a detailed evaluation of their medical histories[4] and those of their mothers along with relevant data on other family members whenever available. All infants included in the study were judged physically normal.

Procedure

For testing, infants were brought to a secluded nursery room where lighting, temperature, and furnishings were constant from day to day. After diapering, the infant was placed in the supine position on the examination crib. We used a standard hospital crib whose sides were kept lowered to 6 inches above the surface of the mattress in order to facilitate observation.

Our procedure consisted of 10 minutes of observation of spontaneous behavior (pretest) during which the observers remained out of view. This period was then followed by a 10-minute standardized test session during which stimulus objects were used to elicit visual pursuit, prehensory, and grasping responses. For the purposes of this report, the prehension-eliciting procedure is most germane. On the basis of several months of pilot work we selected a fringed, multicolored paper party toy as the stimulus object (Figure 1) since it seemed to produce the greatest number of responses in tests of a large number of objects. This object combines a complex contour field with highly contrasting orange, red, and yellow hues. We suspect that these qualities underlie the effectiveness of this stimulus. This speculation is consistent with the findings in the field of visual preferences of human infants (1, 4). The infant's view of the object consists of a red and orange display, circular in form, with a diameter of about 1½ inches. He sees a dark red core, 1 inch square, surrounded by a very irregular outline. Two feathers, one red and one yellow, protrude 1 inch from the sides. We presented the object to the supine infant at three positions for 30 seconds each. Presentations were initiated when the infant's arms were resting on

---

[4] Infants' daily records were screened under the supervision of Drs. P. Wolff and L. Crowell for signs of abnormality using standard medical criteria. Mothers' records were examined for possible genetic pathology and serious complications during pregnancy or delivery.

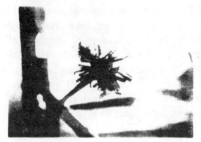

Fig. 1 Stimulus Object

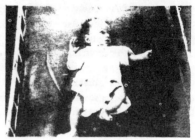

Fig. 2 Tonic Neck Reflex Position

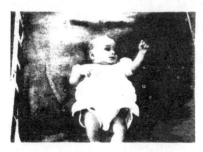

Fig. 3 Hand Regard

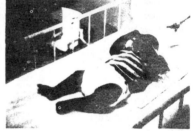

Fig. 4 Hands Clasped at Midline

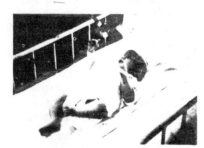

Fig. 5 Both hands raised

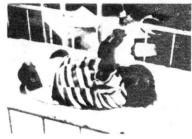

Fig. 6 Oriented Hands Clasped at Midline

the crib surface. The infant's attention is elicited by bringing the stimulus into the infant's line of sight at a distance of about 12 inches and shaking it until the infant fixates it. The infant's head is then led to the appropriate test posture (45° left, 45° right, or midline) by moving the stimulus in the necessary direction while maintaining the infant's attention with renewed shaking of the stimulus when necessary. The object is then brought quickly to within 5 inches of the bridge of the nose and held in a stationary position. Infants over 2½ months of age do not require as much cajoling and the stimulus may be placed at 5 inches immediately. This entire procedure takes no more than 10 seconds with most infants, but occasionally it takes much more time and effort to get young subjects to respond appropriately. The order of presentation was changed from test to test. In certain cases it was necessary to vary the position of the object to determine whether a response was accurately oriented or not. All data were collected by the authors. No infant was tested if he was either ill, drowsy, asleep, or obviously distressed (3, 23). On the average, each infant was tested at weekly intervals. Generally, two observers were present during testing. However, both testing and recording could be handled by a single person.

RESULTS

The Normative Sequence

We found that under our test conditions infants exhibit a relatively orderly developmental sequence which culminates in visually-directed reaching. The following outline, based upon a frequency analysis, describes briefly the spontaneous behaviors and test responses characteristic for each half month interval from 1 through 5 months.

1. 1 to 1½ Months

Pretest observations. The infant lies in the tonic neck reflex position so that his head is fully turned to the side (Figure 2). The hand towards which the eyes are oriented is often in the center of the visual field, but the eyes neither converge on it nor do they adjust to variations in its position. The infant maintains one direction of gaze for prolonged periods. The infant can be made to track a moving object with his head and eyes over an arc of 180° given the proper stimulus conditions. We have obtained reliable responses using a 7½ inch bright red circle against a 14 by 12 inch flat white background as a stimulus. This target is brought into the line of sight of the supine infant at a distance of 12 to 36 inches from the bridge of his nose. Optimal distance at this age is about 24 inches. Attention is elicited by low amplitude, rapid oscillation of the stimulus in the peripheral portion of the visual field. The same motion in the foveal area is ineffective in initiating fixation. Visual pursuit is then induced by moving the target at an approximate speed of 12 inches per second in a semicircular path above the infant's head and in front of his eyes. At this age, pursuit consists of a series of jerky fixations of the red circle which bring its image to the foveal area. As the

81

target continues to move across the field, there is a lag in the following response of the eye until the image again falls on the peripheral region of the retina. At this point, the infant responds with a rapid recentralizing of the image. If the target does not continue its motion or is moving too slowly, and therefore remains in the foveal range for more than a few seconds, the infant's gaze drifts off. We have called this level of response "peripheral pursuit."

Retinoscopic studies (8) indicate that infants have not yet developed flexible accommodative capacities at this age: their focal distance when attending to stimuli between 6 and 16 inches appears to be fixed at about 9 inches. Visual stimuli closer than 7 inches are rarely fixated.

Test responses. In view of the foregoing retinoscopic finding, it is not surprising that the test object fails to elicit the infant's attention. Since the infant's fixed focal distance to near stimuli is approximately 9 inches, the test object at 5 inches produces a badly blurred image on the retina. Usually, however, the infant looks away from the stimulus at this time. When he does attend to the object, he is considerably farsighted (at least three diopters) according to retinoscopic responses. It is clear then that, during this age period, the stimulus is not as effective as it is for older infants whose accommodative capacities are more advanced. This ineffectiveness is probably attributable in large part to loss of the complexity of patterning of the retinal image caused by poor focusing. Occasionally, a brief glance may be directed at the stimulus when it is presented on the side favored by the tonic neck reflex. Presentations on the other side are most always ineffective, since they are generally outside of the infant's field of view, as a result of the tonic neck reflex.

2. 1½ to 2 Months

Pretest observations. The tonic neck reflex is typically present. The infant's eyes occasionally converge on and fixate his own hand (usually the extended hand in the preferred tonic neck reflex posture, Figure 3). The direction of gaze now shifts occasionally to various parts of the visual surround. The responses to the retinoscope indicate that the infant now has the capacity to focus a clear image on the retina when the stimulus is 6 inches above the bridge of the nose. Often, at this age, a new form of visual pursuit is seen. Attention may be elicited in the foveal region using the previously described technique, and tracking is continuous over wide sectors (up to 90°) of the stimulus path. During these periods the response seems to anticipate the motion of the stimulus rather than lagging behind as in peripheral pursuit. We have called this behavior "central" pursuit. This finding is in agreement with Gesell's observations (6).

Test responses. The infant glances at the test object in all presentations. However, sustained fixations are only present on the side of the favored tonic neck reflex. At best, fixation lasts only 5 to 10 seconds. Fixation is judged according to Ling's criteria (18). As Wolff has noted (23), shifts in activity level occur during these periods. At this time such shifts do not follow immediately upon fixation of the object, but appear gradually. Whether the infant becomes more or less active depends on his initial level of behavior. If an infant is alert and inactive, he usually becomes active; whereas if he is active, he becomes less so as he directs his gaze at the stimulus. The latter phenomenon is more common.

3. 2 to 2½ Months

Pretest observations. The tonic neck reflex is still typically present although the head is now only half turned (45°) to the side. In contrast to the previous stages, the infant may shift his gaze rapidly from one part of his surround to another and he rotates his head with comparative ease and rapidity. He now shows a good deal of interest in the examiner. The hand in view in the tonic neck reflex posture is now the object of his attention much of the time that he is awake and alert. The viewed hand may be on the crib surface or held aloft. His eyes now occasionally converge on objects as near as 5 inches from his eyes and central pursuit is usually present. For the first time it is possible to elicit central pursuit of the test object placed as near as 5 inches and moving with a velocity of about 12 inches per second.

Test response. Typically, the infant exhibits immediate and prolonged interest in the stimulus, fixates the object, his activity level shifts, and he makes a swift accurate swipe with the near hand. Usually the object is struck but there is no attempt to grasp since the hand is typically fisted. The probability of a swipe response is greater when the test object is presented on the side of the commonly viewed hand which is the hand extended in the favored tonic neck reflex position.

4. 2½ to 3 Months

Pretest observations. The tonic neck reflex is often present though less frequently than in earlier periods. The head is often near the midline position, and the limbs are usually symmetrically placed. Sustained hand regard continues to be very common. Sustained convergence upon objects as near as 3 inches from the eyes can now be elicited. The infant is more active than at earlier ages. According to retinoscopic examinations, the infant's accommodative capacities are fast approaching adult standards. They differ from the adult in that there is a slightly smaller range of accurate function (5 to 20 inches) and a slower rate of adaptation to the changing stimulus distances.

Test responses. All presentations of the test object result in immediate fixation and an abrupt decrease in activity. Side presentations elicit either swiping behavior as described in the previous age range or else the infant raises the near hand to within an inch or so of the object (unilateral hand raising) and glances repeatedly from object to hand and back (alternating glances).

5. 3 to 3½ Months

Pretest observations. The tonic neck reflex is now rare, and the head is mostly at the midline position. Sustained hand regard is very common, and bilateral arm activity is more frequent than in previous months, with hands clasped together over the midline often present. Occasionally, the glance is directed towards the hands as they approach each other or during their mutual tactual exploration. The infant's accommodative performance is now indistinguishable from that of an adult.

Test responses. The typical response to a side presentation is one or both hands raised with alternating glances from the stimulus to the hand nearest the object. The middle presentation is more likely to elicit bilateral activity such as hands over the midline and clasped (Figure 4), or both hands up (Figure 5), or one hand up and the other to the midline where it clutches the clothing. Here too, alternation of glance from hand to object is common.

6. 3½ to 4 Months

Pretest observations. The tonic neck reflex is now absent. Occasional sustained hand regard continues. Hands clasped over the midline is common, and visual monitoring of their approach and subsequent interplay is usually present.

Test responses. The responses are similar to the previous group with bilateral responses predominating. Hands to the midline and clasped is a favored response at this time even to a side presentation. It is now sometimes combined with a turning of the torso towards the test object (torso orienting).

7. 4 to 4½ Months

Pretest observations. Sustained hand regard is now less common, although examination of hands clasped at the midline is sometimes present. The infant is much more active. The feet are often elevated, and the body is occasionally rotated to the side.

Test responses. Bilateral responses such as hands to midline, both hands up, or one hand up and the other to the midline are now the most common responses to all presentations. These responses are usually accompanied by several alternating glances from the stimulus to one or both hands and back to the stimulus. Torso orientation to the side presentation is now common. At times, the clasped hands are raised and oriented towards the stimulus (Figure 6). Occasionally, one hand will be raised, looked at, and brought slowly to the stimulus while the glance shifts from hand to object repeatedly. When the hand encounters the object it is fumbled at and crudely grasped. This pattern has been described by Piaget (20). Towards the end of this stage, opening of the hand in anticipation of contact with the object is seen.

8. 4½ to 5 Months

Present observations. At this age pretest findings are no different from those obtained during the previous stage.

Test responses. The last stage of this sequence is signified by the appearance of what we call top level reaching.[5] This response is a rapid lifting of

---

[5] Halverson (7) has described the gradual refinement of visually directed reaching from this point on. Subsequent developments, however, concern modifications of the trajectory and posture of the hand rather than new categories of prehensile response.

one hand from out of the visual field to the object. As the hand approaches the object, it opens in anticipation of contact. Hands to the midline with alternating glances and Piaget-type responses are still more likely than top level reaching, but within the next few weeks they drop out rather quickly.

The chronology of 10 response patterns is presented in Table 1. This chronology focuses on the test responses seen most consistently in our subject groups. The columns "Observed In" and "N" indicate that some of the responses are not shown by all subjects. Although 34 subjects were tested, the group size for each response is considerably smaller for several

TABLE 1

Chronology of Responses

Response	Observed In	N	Median and Range of Dates of First Occurrence
			2m — 3m — 4m — 5m — 6m
Swipes at object	13	13	(2:5)
Unilateral hand raising	15	15	(2:17)
Both hands raised	16	18	(2:21)
Alternating glances (hand and object)	18	19	(2:27)
Hands to midline and clasp	15	15	(3:3)
One hand raised with alternating glances, other hand to midline clutching dress	11	19	(3:8)
Torso oriented towards object	15	18	(3:15)
Hands to midline and clasp and oriented towards object	14	19	(4:3)
Piaget-type reach	12	18	(4:10)
Top level reach	14	14	(4:24)
			2m — 3m — 4m — 5m — 6m

85

reasons. First, infants were not available for study for a uniform period of time. All of our subjects were born at the maternity section of the hospital. Usually they were transferred to the children's section at 1 month of age where they remained until they were placed in private homes. Aside from neonatal screening procedures, all tests and observations were performed at the children's section. Some infants arrived from maternity at 1 month of age and stayed through the next 5 or 6 months. Others arrived at the same age and left after a few weeks, and still others arrived as late as 3 months of age, etc. Since we were concerned with the time of emergence of the new forms of behavior, we were obliged to exclude a large number of data because we could not be sure that a late-arriving infant would not have shown the response had we been able to test him earlier.

Another factor which guided us in the analysis of our test protocols was the ease of detection of responses. Each of the 10 items listed is relatively easy to pick out of the diverse behaviors shown by infants and therefore can serve as a developmental index. At times, the presence of a response was questionable. Such data were excluded from the analysis. It is likely therefore that the correct median dates are actually a few days earlier than those charted. A single clear instance of a response was considered sufficient for inclusion in the "observed" column, although multiple instances were by far more common. Another relevant consideration is the limiting effect of weekly testing. Although more frequent testing would have resulted in more accurate data, we felt the added exposure to test conditions might introduce practice effects into our subject groups.

Summary of the Normative Sequence

In summary, then, given the proper object in the proper location and provided that the state of the subject is suitable, our subjects first exhibited object-oriented arm movements at about 2 months of age. The swiping behavior of this stage, though accurate, is not accompanied by attempts at grasping the object; the hand remains fisted throughout the response. From 3 to 4 months of age unilateral arm approaches decrease in favor of bilateral patterns, with hands to the midline and clasped the most common response. Unilateral responses reappear at about 4 months, but the hand is no longer fisted and is not typically brought directly to the object. Rather, the open hand is raised to the vicinity of the object and then brought closer to it as the infant shifts his glance repeatedly from hand to object until the object is crudely grasped. Finally, just prior to 5 months of age, infants begin to reach for and successfully grasp the test object in one quick, direct motion of the hand from out of the visual field.

An Analysis of the Normative Sequence

When one examines the course of development of prehension, it becomes apparent that a number of relatively distinct sensorimotor systems contribute to its growth. These include the visual-motor systems of eye-arm and eye-hand, as well as the tactual-motor system of the hands. These systems seem to develop at different times, partly as a result of varying histories of exposure, and may remain in relative isolation from one another. During the development of prehension these various systems gradually become coordinated into a complex superordinate system which integrates their separate capacities.

During stages 1 and 2 (1 to 2 months), the infant displays several response capacities that are relevant to the ontogeny of prehension. The jerky but coordinated head and eye movements which are seen in *peripheral* visual pursuit are one such capacity. This form of pursuit is an innate coordination since it is present at birth (19). However, another form of pursuit is seen during the second month. The smooth tracking response present in *central* visual pursuit is a more highly refined visual-motor coordination. The path now followed by the eyes appears to anticipate, and thus predict, the future position of a moving target. Whether this response is in fact predictive at this early age remains to be conclusively determined. But this growing capacity of the infant to localize and follow with both his eyes and head is clearly an important prerequisite for the development of visually directed prehension. It should be noted that motion seems to be the stimulus property critical for eliciting attention during this stage.

Arm movements show little organized development at this stage and are limited in the variety of positions that they can assume, in large part because of the influence of the tonic neck reflex. The grasp reflex is present and can be elicited if the palm of the hand encounters a suitable object. But neither of these capacities is yet integrated with the more highly developed visual-motor tracking capacity. Infants of this age do not readily attend to near objects, namely those less than 9 inches distant. Thus, it is not surprising that objects which the infant is able to explore tactually, including his own hands, are not yet visually significant. At this stage, the tactual-motor capacities of the hands remain isolated from the visual-motor ones of the eye and head.

During stages 3 and 4 (2 to 3 months), the isolation of response capacities begins to break down, in part because the infant's eyes can now readily converge and focus on objects that are potentially within his reach. Central pursuit can be elicited from as near as 5 inches. One important consequence of this is that the infant now spends a good deal of time looking at his own hands. In addition, visual interest, sustained fixation, and related shifts in activity level are now readily elicited by a static presentation of the proper stimulus object. This indicates a growing capacity for focusing attention which is no longer exclusively dependent on motion.

In keeping with the above developments, it is at this stage that we see swiping, the first prehensory behavior. The appearance of this behavior indicates the development of a new visual-motor localizing capacity, one which now coordinates not only movements of the eyes and head but also those of the arms. Swiping is highly accurate, although it occasionally overshoots the target. It does not include any attempt at visually controlled grasping. Such grasping would indicate anticipation of contact with the object and is not seen at this stage. Instead, grasping is exclusively a tactually-directed pattern, which remains to be integrated into the growing visual-motor organization of prehension.

The next prehensory response, which develops soon after swiping, is that of raising a hand to within an inch or so of the stationary object followed by a series of alternating glances from object to hand and back. The crude but direct swiping response has been replaced by a more refined behavior. The visual-motor systems of eye-object and eye-hand are now juxtaposed by the infant and seem to be successively compared with each other in some way. This is the kind of behavior that Piaget refers to as the mutual assimilation and accommodation of sensorimotor schemas (24).

During stages 5 and 6 (3 to 4 months), the infant exhibits mutual grasping, a new pattern of spontaneous behavior. This pattern, in which the hands begin to contact and manipulate each other, is particularly important for tactual-motor development. In addition, the visual monitoring of this pattern results in the linking of vision and touch by means of a double feedback system. For the eyes not only see what the hands feel, namely each other, but each hand simultaneously touches and is being actively touched.

In keeping with these developments, hands to midline and clasped is now seen as a test response. This is a tactual-motor response pattern during which the infant fixates the object while the hands grasp each other at the midline. Grasping is thus coming to be related to the now highly developed visual-motor coordination of the head and eyes. At this time, however, grasping is not yet directed towards the external object but remains centered on the tactual interaction of the infant's own hands.

During stages 7 and 8 (4 to 5 months), the infant finally succeeds in integrating the various patterns of response that have developed and coordinating them via their intersection at the object. Thus, alternating glances now become combined with the slow moving of the hand directly to the object which is fumbled at and slowly grasped. The visual-motor schemas of eye-hand and eye-object have now become integrated with the tactual-motor schema of the hand, resulting in the beginnings of visually directed grasping. This pattern has been described by Piaget (20). It is not until the attainment of the highest level of reaching at the end of this stage, however, that one sees the complete integration of the anticipatory grasp into a rapid and direct reach from out of the visual field. Here all the isolated or semi-isolated components of prehensory development come together in the attainment of adult-like reaching just prior to 5 months of age.

The Role of Contact with the Environment

Having made a preliminary analysis of the normative sequence of behaviors, we may proceed to a detailed consideration of the question that originally motivated this study. How can we test for the contribution made by conditions of exposure to the development of prehension? At what stages of growth and in what manner can experimental techniques be applied? Our findings, examined in the light of these questions, yield a projected program of experimental investigation.

Experimental research with both human adults (10, 11, 12, 13, 14, 16) and with animals (15, 21) has strikingly demonstrated the importance of motility for the development and maintenance of visual-motor capacities. This work has shown that the variations in visual stimulation that result from self-produced movements constitute a source of information to the growing nervous system that is required for the proper development of function. Two factors are critical for providing this information. They are certain natural movements of the organism and the presence of stable objects in the environment that can provide sources of visual stimulation that will vary as a consequence of these movements. Deprivation studies with higher infrahuman mammals have shown that, in the absence of either one of these factors, vision does not develop normally (15, 21). No comparable systematic studies of the importance of such factors in the development of human infants are available. However, the complementarity of results between studies of adult rearrangement and of neonatal deprivation in animals (13) leads to specific suggestions as to the conditions of exposure essential for the development of the infant's coordination. For example, in the special case of eye-hand coordination, the work of our laboratory indicates the importance of visual feedback from certain components of motion of the arm, as well as from grosser movements of the body, as in locomotion. How shall we test the applicability of these findings to the development of the human infant? Obviously, we cannot experimentally deprive human infants, but the subjects of the present study are already being reared under conditions that seem to us deficient for optimal development. Thus, we are able to study the effects of systematic additions to the environments of our subjects. Moreover, since our research emphasis is on the importance of the exposure history of the human infant, the fact that our subjects are born and reared under uniform conditions is a distinct advantage. It assures us that previous and current extra-experimental exposure will not be a major source of variability as it might well be under conditions of home-rearing.

The everyday surroundings of our subjects are bland and relatively featureless compared to the average home environment. Moreover, the infants almost always lie in the supine posture which, in comparison to the prone position, is much less conducive to head and trunk motility. Furthermore, the crib matresses have become hollowed out to the point where gross body movements are restricted. We plan to provide a group of these infants with enriched visual surrounds designed to elicit visual-motor responses. In addition, we will place these infants in the prone position for brief periods each day and use plywood supports to flatten the mattress surfaces. These changes should result in significantly greater motility in the presence of stable visible objects. We will assess the effects of such procedures by comparing the sensorimotor capacities of our experimental group with those of a control group reared under currently existing conditions.

We recognize that any effects which may result from the exposure of infants to enriched sensory environments are contingent upon the state of maturation of their neuromuscular mechanisms. We do not, for example, expect visually-directed reaching within the first six weeks of life, when the infant's hands are generally kept fisted and objects within reaching distance are inappropriate for sustained visual fixation. On the other hand, it is quite likely that some aspects of the development of prehension are critically dependent upon prior sensorimotor experience.

A preliminary study has confirmed our suspicion that the onset of sustained hand regard is in part a function of the alternative visual objects present in the infant's environment. For example, under the normal hospital routine where alternative visual objects are at a minimum, the control group of infants began sustained hand viewing at about 2 months of age. In contrast, a pilot group whose cribs were equipped with a variety of objects for viewing failed to exhibit sustained hand regard until 3 months of age. The reason for this marked delay appeared to be the presence of a small mirror placed some 7 inches above the infant's eyes. Invariably, within a week after being placed in the experimental cribs, each infant began to spend most of his waking time staring at his reflection in the mirror. This stimulus virtually monopolized the infants' visual exploratory efforts. This average delay of one month in the appearance of sustained hand regard seems to be clear evidence of the relevance of the visual surround for its development. Since the time of onset can be significantly delayed by a procedure which diverts the infant's attention from his hands, perhaps other procedures designed to direct the infant's attention towards his hands will result in the advanced onset of sustained hand regard. However, the normal hospital environment may already constitute the optimal condition for directing the child's attention to his hands, since there is virtually nothing else for him to look at. If so, our control group should not be considered deprived with respect to the visual requirements underlying the onset of this particular behavior.

Once sustained hand regard appears, swiping at the test object inevitably follows within a few days. On the average, our infants first exhibited swiping responses at 2 months and 3 days of age. We have called this behavior swiping rather than reaching since the hand is kept fisted, thereby precluding successful grasping of the object. Swiping, like visual motor pursuit and fixation, seems to be a stimulus-bound response. This means that the presence of stimuli appropriately designated and located guarantees repeated responses from the infants. The latter half of the path of the swiping response is often viewed by our infants. Moreover, this path is curved rather than direct and entails a rotation of the hand. Precisely this kind of experience has been found necessary for the compensation of errors in reaching caused by the wearing of prism-goggles by human adults (9). We therefore plan to provide our infants with stimulus objects suitably designed to elicit such responses as soon as sustained hand regard appears. We suspect that the increased occurrence of these rotational arm movements, and the feedback stimulation that results, may facilitate the acquisition of eye-hand coordinations in infants. We cannot, however, expect visually-directed prehension to occur at 2½ months of age, even though it seems that we can elicit repeated swiping behavior almost at will. The missing element is the grasp, which is precluded by an innate reflex which keeps the hands fisted, or partially so, until at least 3 months of age.

As the tonic neck reflex drops out at about 3 months of age, the arms are released from their asymmetric posture and tend to move in more similar paths. The inevitable consequences of this development is the mutual discovery of the hands at some point near the middle of the infant's chest. This pattern is initially nonvisual. It is usually several weeks before the infant begins to look at this tactual interplay of his hands. He then spends a great deal of time watching their mutual approach and departure as well as their contacts. Piaget has suggested (20) that this pattern may be conducive to the onset of visually directed prehension of external objects. We have found that this is sometimes the case, but, just as often, infants who exhibit this behavior early are either late in top level reaching or arrive at this stage at about the median age of the group. The prolonged observation of one hand approaching and grasping the other is a virtually innate guarantee of the visual-motor integration of the arm approach and the grasp. On the other hand, since swiping, which appears six weeks earlier, guarantees frequent contact of the hand with the prehensory object, and tactual exploration and the grasp reflex often result in closure, it seems reasonable to assume that integrated prehensory responses would develop through the introduction of suitable external objects at this earlier time. Perhaps it is the absence of such objects that accounts for the 81-day average gap between the onset of swiping responses and the attainment of successful visually-directed reaching seen in our subject group.

In addition to the study of prehension, we plan similar tests of the role of exposure in the development of prerequisite behaviors such as accommodation, convergence, and visual motor pursuit.

REFERENCES

1. BERLYNE, D. The influence of the albedo and complexity of stimuli on visual fixation in the human infant. *Brit. J. Psychol.,* 1958, 49, 315-318.

2. DARWIN, C. *The descent of man.* Modern Library, 1871.

3. ESCALONA, S. The study of individual differences and the problems of state. *J. Amer. Acad. Child Psychiat.,* 1962, 1, 11-37.

4. FANTZ, R. L. A method for studying depth perception in infants under six months of age. *Psychol. Rec.,* 1961, 11, 27-32.

5. GESELL, A., & AMATRUDA, C. *Developmental diagnosis.* Hoeber, 1941.

6. GESELL, A., ILG, F. L., & BULLIS, G. F. *Vision: its development in infant and child.* Hoeber, 1949.

7. HALVERSON, H. M. An experimental study of prehension in infants by means of systematic cinema records. *Genet. Psychol. Monogr.,* 1932, 10, 110-286.

8. HAYNES, H. Retinoscopic studies of human infants. Unpublished manuscript.

9. HEIN, A. Typical and atypical feedback in learning a new coordination. Paper read at Eastern Psychol. Ass., Atlantic City, April, 1959.

10. HELD, R. Shifts in binaural localization after prolonged exposures to atypical combinations of stimuli. *Amer. J. Psychol.*, 1955, 68, 526-548.

11. HELD, R. Exposure-history as a factor in maintaining stability of perception and coordination. *J. nerv. ment. Dis.*, 1961, 132, 26-32.

12. HELD, R. Adaptation to rearrangement and visual-spatial aftereffects. *Psychol. Beiträge*, 1962, 6, 439-450.

13. HELD, R., & BOSSOM, J. Neonatal deprivation and adult rearrangement: complementary techniques for analyzing plastic sensory-motor coordinations. *J. comp. physiol. Psychol.*, 1961, 54, 33-37.

14. HELD, R., & HEIN, A. Adaptation of disarranged hand-eye coordinations contingent upon reafferent stimulation. *Percept. mot. Skills*, 1958, 8, 87-90.

15. HELD, R., & HEIN, A. Movement-produced stimulation in the development of visually-guided behavior. *J. comp. physiol. Psychol.*, 1963, 56, 872-876.

16. HELD, R., & SCHLANK, M. Adaptation to optically-increased distance of the hand from the eye by reafferent stimulation. *Amer. J. Psychol.*, 1959, 72, 603-605.

17. JONES, F. W. *Arboreal man.* London: E. Arnold, 1916.

18. LING, B. A genetic study of sustained visual fixation and associated behavior in the human infant from birth to six months. *J. genet. Psychol.*, 1942, 61, 227-277.

19. PEIPER, A. *Die Eigenart der Kindlichen Hirntätigkeit.* (2nd ed.) Leipzig: Thieme, 1956.

20. PIAGET, J. *The origins of intelligence in children.* (2nd ed.) International Universities Press, 1952.

21. RIESEN, A. H. Plasticity of behavior: psychological series. In H. Harlow and C. Woolsey (Eds.), *Biological and biochemical bases of behavior.* Univer. of Wisconsin Press, 1958. Pp. 425-450.

22. RIESEN, A. H. Stimulation as a requirement for growth and function in behavioral development. In D. W. Fiske and S. R. Maddi (Eds.), *Functions of varied experience.* Dorsey Press, 1961. Pp. 57-80.

23. WOLFF, P. H. Observations on newborn infants. *Psychosom. Med.*, 1959, 21, 110-118.

24. WOLFF, P. H. The developmental psychologies of Jean Piaget and psychoanalysis. *Psychol. Issues*, 1960, 2, 1-181.

AMPLITUDE, POSITION, TIMING AND VELOCITY AS CUES IN REPRODUCTION OF MOVEMENT[1]

RONALD G. MARTENIUK, KENNETH W. SHIELDS, SHARON CAMPBELL

Summary.—In three experiments the method of average error was used to study the reproductions of amplitudes of standard horizontal arm movements ranging from 45° to 125°. Response sensitivity, in terms of mean difference limens and absolute errors, was relatively precise and constant over the range of movement. However, constant errors exhibited a definite trend in that small movements were constantly overestimated and large ones were underestimated. It was also found that the starting and terminal positions of a movement were important cues in movement reproduction, whereas timing ability and movement velocity seemed unrelated to accuracy.

The present study was designed to provide some fundamental data on the sensitivity of the kinesthetic system. Kinesthesis is the sensory modality concerned with the conscious perception of movement and orientation of the parts of the body with respect to each other and with respect to the body as a whole (Howard & Templeton, 1966). Recent interest in kinesthesis has been centered around the role that this sense might play in providing information for the control of movement. More specifically kinesthesis has been included in models of human performance and has been seen as an important segment in the closed-loop control of movement (Keele, 1968; Adams, 1968, 1971; Marteniuk, 1971). However, very little evidence has been accumulated on the basic properties of this sense and especially on to what cues this system is sensitive.

The present study consisted of three separate experiments. The first, while dealing with the accuracy of active kinesthesis, also dealt with the question of whether the sensitivity of this system is a constant over the range of movement studied. The second experiment was designed to determine the relative importance of position and movement cues to the reproduction of movement. Finally, the third experiment provided information as to whether timing ability and arm velocity were used as cues.

GENERAL METHOD

Subjects

In total, 52 right-handed male university students, ranging in age from 19 to 35 yr. of age, participated as *S*s. There were three separate experiments with 10, 18, and 24 different *S*s, respectively.

Apparatus

The movement apparatus consisted of a half-circle of masonite board with

---

[1]This study was supported in part by the National Research Council of Canada.

PERCEPTUAL MOTOR SKILLS, 1972, Vol. 35, pp. 51-58.

an 180° arc, calibrated in ½°, drawn on it. A lever with a pointer was attached to a frictionless pivot at the center of the arc. S moved the lever by means of a handle which could be adjusted along the length of the lever.

Procedure

For all experiments a common procedure was used. Before entering the laboratory each S was stripped to the waist and blindfolded. For those conditions which involved reproduction of movement S was then placed before the apparatus and the handle of the lever was adjusted so that when S grasped it, his elbow was directly over the pivot of the lever. The starting position for movements was standardized over Ss, with the lever at the 30° point on the apparatus. From this point the procedure differed depending in what experiment and condition S was in. However, basically the procedure was for E to present a standard movement to S either by having S actively move the lever to a physical stop or by E moving the lever in a similar manner so that S's arm was moved passively. This movement constituted the standard movement. S or E, depending on whether it was an active or passive condition, then returned the lever to the starting position and S was then required actively to reproduce the movement as accurately as possible without the aid of the stop. The algebraic error associated with the reproduction was then recorded to the nearest half degree. The presentation of the standard and its reproduction was called a trial.

For the one experiment that involved time reproduction, the standard time to be reproduced was presented to the blindfolded S through the use of an interval timer and two switches. E started the time interval by closing the switch, which produced a loud click, and the interval timer, after a preset interval, opened the second switch which again produced a loud click. S was then required to reproduce the interval between the two clicks by pressing a button he held in his left hand to start the interval (which also started a clock) and ending the interval by pressing a button in his right hand which stopped the clock. The algebraic error associated with the time reproduction was recorded to the nearest millisecond.

For all movement and time trials the time between trials was kept as close to 2 sec. as was possible. Other controls employed consisted of a pre-training session so that Ss could become familiar with the task and with the required velocity of movement which was approximately 1 sec. for every 30°.

EXPERIMENT 1

Experimental Design

In this experiment there were three conditions and they differed only in the length of standard movement employed. These standards were 45°, 90°, and 125°.

Each of the 10 Ss was given a total of 100 trials per standard where the trials were presented in blocks of 20 with a 1-min. rest between blocks and a 5-min. rest between standards. The order in which the 10 Ss performed the three conditions was controlled so that each condition was encountered first, second, and third by Ss approximately an equal number of times.

Results

The mean difference limens (DLs) for the 100 trials taken as 0.6745 $\times$ SD, where SD is the standard deviation of a number of error scores for a S (Woodworth & Schlosberg, 1956), were 1.95°, 2.20°, and 2.13° for the standards of 45°, 90° and 125°, respectively. An analysis of variance indicated that these DLs were not statistically different from each other. However, the mean constant errors (CEs), or algebraic errors, for the same three standards did produce a significant F. The Scheffe technique indicated that only the difference between the 45° standard (CE = 1.05°) and the 90° standard (−0.69°) were different from one another with the CE of the 125° standard being −0.07°. The analysis of the mean absolute errors (AEs), where the sign of the error was disregarded, indicated these means to be statistically equal. AEs for the 45°, 90° and 125° standards were 2.66°, 2.92° and 2.94°.

Discussion

The above results indicated that sensitivity over a 125° range was not only relatively precise but also constant in that small and homogeneous DLs were obtained for standards of 45°, 90°, and 125° in each of the two experiments. This finding was reinforced when it was found that the AEs over the three standards in each experiment did not differ significantly from each other. These data are supported by the work of Caldwell and Herbert (1956) who reported that response variability for their Ss was relatively constant over the 90° range of movement for a horizontal arm-positioning task. In another study Caldwell (1956) found that response variability was less at the extremes of a 90° arm movement but attributed this finding to anchoring effects. Thus, in light of the evidence on active movement of the arm, it seems that the type of kinesthetic mechanism involved in discrimination of movement is a qualitative receptor mechanism. In other words, any increase in magnitude of movement activates different populations of receptors in the joint capsule. This line of reasoning is supported by evidence presented in the works of Smith (1969), Williams (1969), and Mountcastle and Powell (1959) where they show that at both the joint-receptor level and cortical level, specific cells correspond to specific limb positions.

In terms of mean CEs, the results indicated that some variation occurred that was attributable to the amplitude of the standard movement. These findings, in terms of relative accuracy, are in agreement with previous research by Cohen (1958) who reported a mean error of 3 cm. for an arm-positioning task in the frontal plane. Also, Caldwell and Herbert (1956) reported CEs ranging from +0.50 to −2.9° for an arm-positioning task ranging from 0° to 90°, while Lloyd and Caldwell (1956) reported slightly larger CEs for a leg-positioning task. One finding of the above experiment that was similar to the studies of Caldwell and Herbert (1956) and Lloyd and Caldwell (1956) was the fact that positive CEs were obtained for relatively short movements and for longer movements increasingly negative CEs occurred.

EXPERIMENT 2

Experimental Conditions and Design

To determine what influence position cues had on the ability to reproduce a movement three experimental conditions were employed. Condition 1 involved reproducing a 90° movement in an identical manner to the method employed in Exp. 1. For this particular experiment it can be noted that this movement entailed both position and active movement cues.

In Condition 2 each trial was initiated by E who moved S's positioning lever while S relaxed his arm as it moved with the lever. E attempted to destroy all movement cues by moving the lever through a series of short and long overlapping cues before the lever was stopped at the 90° standard position. At this time E said "standard" to S and held the lever at this position for approximately 2 sec. E then returned the lever to the starting position in a manner similar to which the lever had been brought to the standard position. S then attempted to reproduce actively the standard position. Thus this condition involved position cues but no movement cues.

Condition 3 was an attempt to isolate the effect of active-movement cues from position cues. To accomplish this S performed in a similar manner as in Condition 1 of this experiment except that while he was returning the lever from the stopper, which had designated the amplitude of the standard movement, a second stopper was randomly placed at positions corresponding to 13°, 18°, and 23° from the original starting position (i.e., 0°). This block stopped the lever and S then attempted to reproduce the amplitude of the movement involved in travelling to the block at 90°. Thus, if the returning lever had been stopped at 13°, a correct reproduction would have been made to 103°.

In this experiment 18 Ss performed 15 trials in each of the three conditions. Each S was systematically assigned to one of the six possible orders in which the three conditions could be performed. In this way there were three Ss per order and the effect due to order could be examined.

Results

The data from the three conditions are given in Table 1. For the DL data a significant F from the analysis of variance was obtained. Scheffe's test indicated that the DL from Condition 1, active movement with position cues, was significantly smaller than either of the other two conditions.

In terms of CE a significant over-all F was again achieved and Scheffe's test

TABLE 1

POSITION VS MOVEMENT CUES IN ACCURACY OF MOVEMENT REPRODUCTION

Score	Condition 1 active movement with positioning	Condition 2 passive movement with positioning	Condition 3 active movement with no positioning
Difference limen	3.324°	4.936°	5.442°
Constant error	—0.428°	+1.443°	—3.424°
Absolute error	3.446°	4.550°	6.376°

Note.—See text for description of different conditions.

96

showed that the differences between Condition 3, active movement with no position cues, and the other two conditions were significant. For AE the same pattern of significant differences occurred, with Condition 3 producing significantly larger AEs than both Conditions 1 and 2.

For the above data, the order in which the conditions were performed had no effect on size of the scores as evidenced by nonsignificant F ratios for the main effect of order.

Discussion

In the above experiment, Condition 1 served as a control where cues from active movement and position, i.e., the starting position and the termination point of the standard movement, were both present. Condition 2 used passive movement where it was assumed that kinesthetic cues from movement amplitude would be minimal or absent (Keele, 1968; Lloyd & Caldwell, 1956) and that there would be no cues from the motor command to the muscles (Keele, 1968). Thus, the only cues available to S would be those derived from the starting position of the limb and the position of the limb as it was held at the end point of the standard movement. Finally, Condition 3 was designed to determine what influence the starting position for a movement had on its reproduction. In this condition only amplitude cues could be used by Ss to make their reproduction of movement.

The results indicated that, without starting-position or end-position cues (Condition 3), Ss were significantly less accurate in terms of the DL, CE and AE, than when they were present (Condition 1). When only active-movement cues were eliminated (Condition 2) performance in general was better than Condition 3 but not as good as in Condition 1. These results are similar to those of Posner (1967) where he found that over-all accuracy was greater when reproduction was from the same starting position. Thus, the above results suggest that active-movement cues *per se* do not provide sufficient information for accurate reproduction of movement. Most definitely other important cues are derived from the starting position of the movement as well as the position of the limb at the end point of the movement.

EXPERIMENT 3

Experimental Conditions and Design

Half of this experiment was a replication of Exp. 1 with the exception that instead of S performing 100 trials for each of the three standard movements, 45°, 90°, and 120°, only 15 trials were attempted. In addition, microswitches placed at the starting position and 10° short of each standard enabled E to record the time in msec. that it took S to move the lever during both the presentation of the standard movement and its reproduction.

The second half of this experiment involved the same Ss attempting to reproduce standard time intervals of 1, 3, and 5 sec. Again 15 trials per standard were given to each S. Of the 24 Ss in this experiment 12 performed the movement conditions first while the other 12 completed the timing conditions first. The order effect, within both the timing and movement conditions, was balanced across Ss.

Results

The first half of this experiment served as a replication of Exp. 1. Table 2 presents these results and, by comparing these with data of Exp. 1, it can be seen that the two experiments produced relatively similar results. As in Exp. 1 there were no significant differences among the three standards in Exp. 3 for both the DLs and AEs. For CE the same trend of overshooting the shortest standard and undershooting the longest standard was evident in both experiments. For Exp. 3 and 45° CE was significantly different from the 90° CE, all other differences among the CEs of the three standards being nonsignificant.

TABLE 2

ACCURACY OF MOVEMENT REPRODUCTION FOR THREE STANDARD MOVEMENTS

Score	Standard Movement		
	45°	90°	125°
Difference limen	2.41°	2.31°	2.19°
Constant error	1.51°	0.85°	−0.34°
Absolute error	3.69°	3.60°	2.93°

It is interesting to note that the trend in CEs, i.e., a positive CE for the short standard and a negative CE for the long standard which could be taken as an effect due to regression toward the mean standard, was not an artifact of the order in which the standards were performed since the F for the order effect was less than 1.00. The order effect was also nonsignificant for the DLs and AEs.

The results from the second half of Exp. 3, reproduction of intervals of time, are presented in Table 3. The over-all F for differences among standards was significant for the DLs, CEs, and AEs. The only significant difference for both the DLs and CEs was the difference between the 1-sec. and 5-sec. standards. For AE the 1-sec. standard was significantly different from both the 3-sec. and 5-sec. standards.

To determine if there was any relationship between the ability to discriminate movement and the ability to discriminate time the DLs from the standard movements were correlated with the DLs for time. In general, the correlations

TABLE 3

ACCURACY OF TIME REPRODUCTION (SEC.) FOR THREE STANDARD TIMES

Score	Standard Time		
	1 sec.	3 sec.	5 sec.
Difference limen	0.16	0.23	0.29
Constant error	−0.005	0.075	0.197
Absolute error	0.246	0.415	0.519

were low with the highest correlation, 0.46, accounting for less than 23% of the variance between the two variables. The average of the nine possible correlations between the three movement conditions and the three time conditions was 0.18.

Also of interest were the correlations between the time taken for a movement to the physical stop when S was presented a standard movement and the time taken for the movement when reproducing that standard. These correlations, based on scores representing an average of 15 trials, were 0.91, 0.74, and 0.85 sec. for the 45°, 90°, and 125° standards respectively. Evidently Ss used the same relative velocity of movement when reproducing a movement as they had when previously being presented with the standard. Other correlations of interest were those between the DLs, CEs, and AEs for the three standard movements and the average velocity of the standard and reproduction movements for the 15 trials of each standard. In all cases these correlations were very low, ranging from -0.26 to $+0.43$ and indicating that velocity of movement had relatively little influence on the accuracy of that movement.

Discussion

This experiment was, in essence, a replication of Exp. 1 and the results indicated that there was a good deal of similarity between these two experiments in terms of DLs, CEs, and AEs for each of the three lengths of movement. Thus, it appears that the particular task used in the present experiments produces relatively consistent results over different groups of Ss.

In terms of the other results from Exp. 3, position cues seemed to influence reproduction of accuracy of movement to a considerable extent but the same was not found for the ability to discriminate time. The results indicated that timing accuracy, as measured by the DL of time reproduction, correlated rather poorly with accuracy of movement. The same results were obtained for velocity of movement in that the correlations of this variable with accuracy of movement were also very low and tended to be near zero. Thus, it appears that at least for the conditions of the present study, timing ability and velocity of movement play a rather small role in reproduction of movement.

REFERENCES

ADAMS, J. A. Response feedback and learning. *Psychological Bulletin,* 1968, 70, 486-504.

ADAMS, J. A. A closed-loop theory of motor learning. *Journal of Motor Behavior,* 1971, 3, 111-150.

CALDWELL, L. A. The accuracy of constant angular displacement of the arm in the horizontal plane as influenced by the direction and locus of the primary adjustive movement. *USA MRL Rep.,* 1956, Tech. Rep. 233.

CALDWELL, L. A., & HERBERT, M. J. The judgment of angular positions in the horizontal plane on the basis of kinesthetic cues. *USA MRL Rep.,* 1956, Tech. Rep. 216.

COHEN, L. A. Analysis of position sense in the human shoulder. *Journal of Neurophysiology,* 1958, 21, 560-562.

HOWARD, I. P., & TEMPLETON, W. B. *Human spatial orientation.* London: Wiley, 1966.

KEELE, S. W. Movement control in skilled motor behavior. *Psychological Bulletin,* 1968, 70, 387-403.

LLOYD, A. J., & CALDWELL, L. S. Accuracy of active and passive positioning of the leg on the basis of kinesthetic cues. *Journal of Comparative Physiology and Psychology,* 1956, 9, 102-106.

MARTENIUK, R. G. An informational analysis of active kinesthesis as measured by amplitude of movement. *Journal of Motor Behavior,* 1971, 3, 69-77.

MOUNTCASTLE, V. B., & POWELL, P. S. Central nervous mechanism subserving positioning sense and kinesthesis. *Johns Hopkins Hospital Bulletin,* 1959, 108, 173-200.

POSNER, N. I. Characteristics of visual and kinesthetic memory codes. *Journal of Experimental Psychology,* 1967, 73, 103-107.

SMITH, J. L. Kinesthesis: a model for movement feedback. In R. C. Brown & B. J. Cratty (Eds.), *New perspectives of man in action.* Englewood Cliffs, N. J.: Prentice-Hall, 1969. Pp. 31-50.

WILLIAMS, H. G. Neurological concepts and perceptual motor behavior. In R. C. Brown & B. J. Cratty (Eds.), *New perspectives of man in action.* Englewood Cliffs, N. J.: Prentice-Hall, 1969. Pp. 51-73.

WOODWORTH, R. S., & SCHLOSBERG, H. *Experimental psychology.* New York: Holt, Rinehart & Winston, 1956.

PART IV

EFFECTING VOLUNTARY CONTROL OVER
VISCERAL AND GLANDULAR RESPONSES

Control and Training of Individual Motor Units

J. V. BASMAJIAN

Abstract. *Experiments clearly demonstrate that with the help of auditory and visual cues man can single out motor units and control their isolated contractions. Experiments on the training of this control, interpreted as the training of descending pathways to single anterior horn cells, provide a new glimpse of the fineness of conscious motor controls. After training, subjects can recall into activity different single motor units by an effort of will while inhibiting the activity of neighbors. Some learn such exquisite control that they soon can produce rhythms of contraction in one unit, imitating drum rolls, etc. The quality of control over individual anterior horn cells may determine rates of learning.*

It is a commonplace observation that very gentle contractions of skeletal muscles recruit only a few motor units and that, on relaxation, human beings can promptly repress all neuromuscular activity in large areas under voluntary control (1). However, little attention has been paid to the fine voluntary control of individual motor units. In 1960 Harrison and Mortensen (2) reported that subjects were able to maintain isolated activity of several different motor units in the tibialis anterior as recorded from surface electrodes and confirmed by needle electrodes. The implications of this finding led to an intensive systematic investigation with special indwelling electrodes.

By definition, a motor unit includes a spinal anterior horn cell, its axon, and all the muscle fibers on which the terminal branches of the axon end (Fig. 1). This motor unit "fires" when an impulse reaches the muscle fibers, the response being a brief twitch. The electrical potential accompanying the twitch is now well documented. The twitch frequency has an upper limit of about 50 per second. With indwelling electrodes, individual motor units are identifiable by their individual shapes; these remain relatively constant unless the electrodes are shifted.

The subjects of these experiments were provided with two modalities of "proprioception" that they normally lack, namely, they heard their motor unit potentials and saw them on monitors. The subjects were 16 normal persons ranging in age from 20 to 55. All but five were under 24 and only one was female.

The main muscle tested in all subjects was the right abductor pollicis brevis (Fig. 2). In two subjects the tibialis anterior was also tested; in another, the biceps brachii and the extensor digitorum longus were tested on other occasions. The recording and monitoring apparatus is illustrated in Fig. 2.

The indwelling electrodes used have

SCIENCE, 1963, Vol. 141, pp. 440-441.

already been described in detail (3). They are nylon-insulated Karma alloy wires 0.025 mm in diameter, which are introduced into the muscle as a pair by means of a hypodermic needle that is immediately withdrawn. In the case of a small muscle like the abductor pollicis brevis, the activity of all its motor units are probably detected while the fascial coat of the muscle isolates the pick-up to this muscle alone.

After placement and connection of the electrodes, the subjects spent 5 to 10 minutes becoming familiar with the response of the electromyograph to a range of movements and postures. They were invariably amazed at the responsiveness to even the slightest effort. Then they began learning how to maintain very slight contractions, which were apparent to themselves only through the response of the apparatus. This led to increasingly more demanding effort involving many procedures intended to reveal both their natural talent in controlling individual motor units and their skill in learning and retaining tricks with such units. Individual units were identified by the characteristics of their potentials which show considerable difference on the oscilloscope and, to a lesser extent, on the loudspeaker. Film recordings of potentials were made for confirmation (Fig. 3).

Generally, experiments on one muscle were limited to about half a day. Within 15 to 30 minutes all subjects had achieved notably better willful control over gentle contractions. In this time almost all had learned to relax the whole muscle instantaneously on command and to recruit the activity of a single motor unit, keeping it active for as many minutes as desired. A few had difficulty maintaining the activity of such a unit, or in recruiting more units.

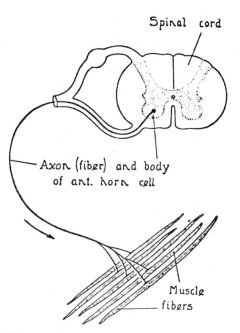

Fig. 1. Diagram of a motor unit of skeletal muscle.

No relationship was obvious to age, manual dexterity, or anything that might have been invoked as an underlying explanation of the differences in performance. Two of the apparently most dexterous persons performed only moderately well. The youngest persons were among both the worst and the best performers.. General personality traits did not seem to matter.

After about 30 minutes the subject was required to learn how to repress the first motor unit he had become familiar with and to recruit another one. Most subjects were able to do this and gain mastery of the new unit in a matter of minutes; only one subject required more than 15 minutes. More than half of the subjects could repeat the performance with a third new unit within a few minutes. A few subjects could recruit a fourth or a fifth isolated unit. The

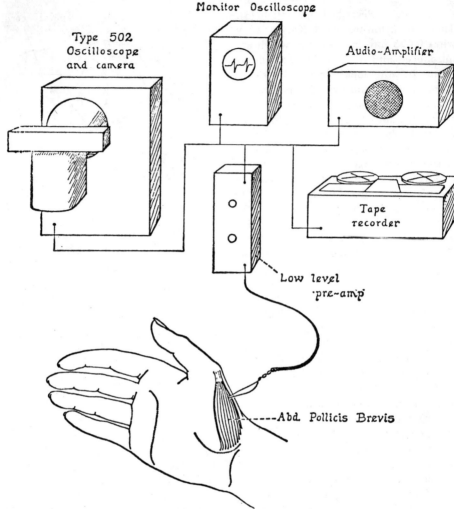

Fig. 2. Technique of recording from abductor pollicis brevis.

next problem facing a subject was to recruit, unerringly and in isolation, the several units over which he had gained control.

Here there was a considerable variation in skill. About one in four could respond easily to the command for isolated contractions of any of three units. About half the subjects displayed much less skill in this regard, even after several hours and even though they may have learned other bizarre tricks. Several subjects had particular difficulty in recruiting the asked-for units. They groped around in their conscious efforts to find them and sometimes, it seemed, only succeeded by accident.

The subjects with the finest control were then trained to learn various tricks. Several were tested for their powers of recalling specific units into activity in the *absence* of the aural and

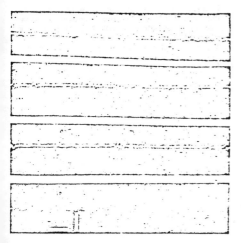

Fig. 3. Electromyograms of potentials from motor units, *A*, *B*, and *C*, and of a weak-to-moderate contraction (tracing *D*) in the abductor pollicis brevis of one subject. Calibrations lines: 25 msec and 200 μv.

visual feedbacks which were so important to most of the subjects. Three subjects could recall units voluntarily under these handicaps, but they were unable to explain how they could do it.

Other tests showed that in all subjects the aural feedback is more useful than the visual display on the cathode ray tube monitor. The latter served only a subsidiary purpose.

After 60 to 90 minutes, most of the subjects were tested and trained in the production of specific rhythms. Almost all could reduce and increase the frequency of a well-controlled unit. It soon became apparent that motor units do not have a single characteristic frequency. Rather, they have an individual maximum rate below which their firing can be greatly slowed and single isolated contractions can be produced. Above the maximum rate that is characteristic for a specific unit, overflow

takes place and other motor units are recruited.

Subjects learned to control units so that they could produce various rhythms. Almost all the subjects in the later experiments who were asked to try these (10 of 11) succeeded. Various gallop rhythms, drum-beat rhythms, doublets, and roll effects were produced and recorded (4).

The experiments reported above suggest that pathways from the cerebral cortex can be made to stimulate single anterior horn cells while neighboring anterior horn cells remain dormant or are depressed. Although the skills learned in these experiments depended on aural and visual feedbacks from muscles, the controls are learned so quickly, are so exquisite, and are so well retained after the feedbacks are eliminated in some subjects, that one must not dismiss them as tricks. The underlying mechanisms seem to involve active suppression of neighboring anterior horn cells.

A number of obvious problems emerge from the differences in the rates of learning of motor unit skills by different subjects. New but limited studies by Harrison (5) suggest that accomplished athletes have no better control than other subjects over their motor units. Future studies to ascertain the relation of rates of motor unit learning to dexterity, special abilities, and techniques of teaching motor skills are called for.

The extremely fine ability to adjust the rate of firing of individual motor units is a novel concept. Above a characteristic frequency, which varies from cell to cell, overflow to neighbors occurs. Detailed studies of these characteristics should expose some of the underlying control mechanism in the spinal cord (6).

References and Notes

1. J. V. Basmajian, *Muscles Alive: Their Functions Revealed by Electromyography* (Williams and Wilkins, Baltimore, 1962), p. 7.
2. V. F. Harrison and O. A. Mortensen (abstract), *Anat. Record*, 136, 207 (1960); 144, 109 (1962).
3. J. V. Basmajian and G. Stecko, *J. Appl. Physiol.* 17, 849 (1962).
4. Excerpts of tape recordings were played to the annual meeting of the American Association of Anatomists, April 1963, as part of a paper of mine.
5. V. F. Harrison (abstract), *Anat. Record*, 145, 237 (1963).
6. Supported by grants from the Muscular Dystrophy Association of Canada and the Medical Research Council of Canada. Glenn Shine provided technical assistance.

FEEDBACK-INDUCED MUSCLE RELAXATION: APPLICATION TO TENSION HEADACHE*

THOMAS BUDZYNSKI, JOHANN STOYVA and CHARLES ADLER

Summary—This paper describes a technique for producing deep muscle relaxation by means of an information feedback technique—the subject hears a tone with a frequency proportional to the EMG level of the muscle being monitored. The new technique was applied to several tension headache patients—the first five individuals available for the study. With this 'bio-feedback' training in relaxation, the patients not only learned to produce low frontalis EMG levels but showed subsequent reductions in headache activity.

Sources in the medical literature are fairly well agreed that the tension headache (or muscle contraction headache) is associated with sustained contraction of the scalp and neck muscles (Ostfeld, 1962; Wolff, 1963; Martin, 1966). Therefore we decided to observe whether a technique for training individuals in deep muscle relaxation which we recently developed in our laboratory (Budzynski and Stoyva, 1969) could be used to alleviate this disorder. This technique, and the basic instrumentation it requires, will be described first. Then we will discuss its application to five patients with tension headache.

INSTRUMENTATION

The basic function of the instrumentation (see Fig. 1) is to assist subjects in reaching deep levels of muscle relaxation by means of analog information feedback; that is, subjects hear a tone with a frequency proportional to the electromyographic (EMG) activity in the relevant muscle group. If there is a high level of EMG activity in the muscle being monitored, the tone is high pitched; as EMG activity decreases, the tone decreases in frequency. Feedback tone thus tracks the fluctuating level of EMG activity in the muscle.

The subject, who has EMG electrodes applied to the skin surface over a particular muscle (e.g. frontalis or forearm extensor), has to keep the tone low by relaxing that muscle. As he gradually gets better at doing this, the loop gain of the feedback system is increased, thus requiring him to maintain a lower EMG level in order to hear a low tone. The response of deep muscle relaxation is increased by increasing the difficulty of the task in a series of finely graded steps.

The sequence of events in the feedback system is as follows: first, a Grass P15 a.c. preamplifier is used to amplify (G = 1000) the bioelectric signal generated in the muscle. The amplified EMG signal is then both quantified and converted into a feedback signal by the BIFS (Bioelectric Information Feedback System). This unit, which is compatible with most a.c. polygraph amplifiers, further amplifies the EMG signal, then filters, rectifies and integrates it. The resulting fluctuating d.c. signal drives a voltage-controlled-oscillator which converts the fluctuating d.c. signal into an a.c. signal (a sine

*Paper presented at the Ninth Annual Meeting of the Society for Psychophysiological Research, Monterey, California, October, 1969.

We are most grateful to Gordon Globus, Department of Psychiatry, University of California, Irvine, for drawing our attention to the etiology of tension headache, and to Catherine McKay for technical assistance.

Supported by the National Institutes of Mental Health, Grant Number MH-15596, and Research Scientist Development Award, Grant Number KO1-MH-43361-01.

JOURNAL OF BEHAVIOR THERAPY AND EXPERIMENTAL PSYCHIATRY, 1970, vol. 1, pp. 205-211.

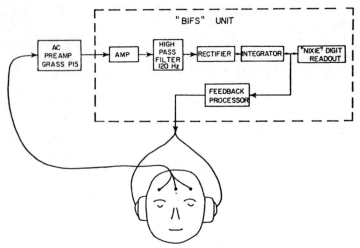

FIG. 1. Functional diagram: EMG information feedback.

wave) of varying frequency. This is conveyed through headphones to the subject as a constant volume tone which varies in frequency as muscle EMG changes. In short, this system allows him to 'hear' his own muscle activity.

In measuring the EMG from a relaxed muscle it is important to use a low noise a.c. amplifier which has high input impedance and high common mode rejection (if it has a differential input). Such an amplifier is necessary to establish a suitable signal-to-noise ratio for the low level EMG signal generated by relaxed muscles. The bandwidth of the amplifier is restricted in order to reduce noise and to eliminate artifact from other higher level bioelectric signals such as EKG and EEG. In this study the bandwidth was 120–1000 Hz.

A precise quantification of minute-by-minute EMG levels is provided by a constant reset level integration technique (Shaw, 1967) which is available to the experimenter as a four digit NIXIE tube readout. The integration process is such that the final figure which has accumulated on the readout panel (and is held for 20 sec) represents the average level of EMG activity in microvolts peak-to-peak for that particular

1-min trial. Thus, over a series of 1-min trials, EMG levels might be 11·20, 10·54, 8·23, 8·66, 6·77 and 6·42 μV for six consecutive trials. The resulting data, minute-by-minute EMG levels, are extremely useful in studying human dynamics in a feedback loop.

It will be noted that this 'bio-feedback training' system directly incorporates two major characteristics of operant conditioning—immediate knowledge of results and the gradual shaping of responses.

PROCEDURE

Since the procedure was essentially the same for each of the five patients, the training technique will be described in detail only for the very first patient trained in bio-feedback muscle relaxation.

This patient was a 29-year-old research technician, married and without children. Since the age of nine she had regularly suffered from tension headaches of varying intensity. These were bilateral, dull, aching frontal headaches, gradual in onset, beginning in the morning and generally lasting all day—a classical tension headache picture. The patient was first given a thorough medical examination by a collaborating psychiatric resident physician, in order to rule out the possibility of neurological and other organic disorders and to confirm the diagnosis of tension headache. Training in bio-feedback muscle relaxation was then begun.

Since tension headache is produced by sustained contraction of the neck and scalp muscles it was decided to use the frontalis (forehead) muscle in the feedback loop, i.e. patients would receive feedback from muscle action potentials generated in the forehead area. An earlier study (Budzynski and Stoyva, 1969) had indicated that subjects can learn to lower frontalis EMG levels much more effectively with bio-feedback training than without it. The subjects in this study had also reported that the deep muscle relaxation seemed to generalize to other muscles of the body, especially the upper body and head musculature.

For a particular training session, the procedure was as follows: EMG surface electrodes were placed 1 in. above each eyebrow and spaced 4 in. apart on the patient's forehead. One reference electrode was placed in the center of the forehead. Electrode resistances were 10,000 ohms or less. The patient reclined on a couch in a dimly-lighted, electrically shielded room.

During her first two sessions in the laboratory, she practised relaxing *without* the benefit of any feedback. Both times frontalis EMG levels were recorded for twenty trials. As the investigators had expected, her EMG levels were exceptionally high—nearly twice the usual baseline values for normal subjects previously run in this laboratory.

In the bio-feedback training sessions, which began with her third visit to the laboratory, she heard low-pitched tones whenever her frontalis muscle was relatively relaxed, and higher-pitched tones whenever the frontalis was not relaxed. She was told that the tone would follow her tension level and that she should try to keep the tone low in pitch. An important aspect of the training was the 'shaping' procedure—

accomplished by varying the gain of the feedback loop. As she progressed—by relaxing the frontalis—the gain of the feedback loop was gradually increased, making the task more difficult since she was obliged progressively to decrease her level of EMG activity in order to keep the feedback tone at low frequencies. The patient's response was thus being 'shaped' in the sense that the gain was carefully adjusted to maintain performance at the low tone level approximately 80 per cent of the time. (This level was found in our pilot studies not to produce frustration and yet allow learning to occur.)

The patient received two or three 30-min feedback training sessions per week, and worked at bringing her frontalis EMG to low levels. Over the weeks, as she grew more proficient at relaxing, an increasing number of silent trials were interspersed among the feedback trials. These silent trials were designed to help her maintain the relaxation response even in the absence of the feedback tone.

She was encouraged to practice relaxation training at home at least once a day. Each of the other four patients was similarly encouraged to do the home training since the investigators felt that the ability to produce the relaxation response outside the laboratory was essential if the patients were to be enabled to prevent or alleviate their tension headaches in everyday life.

The patient also had to keep a daily record of her headaches. From her first baseline day, she was asked to fill out daily headache charts. These charts were little trouble for her to complete, and proved to be extremely useful in the quantification of headache activity. The charts were small (3 by 5 in.) cards with a grid and a horizontal and vertical scale. The vertical scale represented headache intensity from 0 to 5, with 5 indicating a very intense headache. On the horizontal axis was a time scale—hours of the day—beginning at 6 a.m. on the left and ending at 5 a.m. on the right. The subject plotted one point for each waking hour.

Training time varied from 4 weeks to 2 months depending upon the level of headache activity in the individual patients.

INDIVIDUAL RESULTS

Patient 1

An analysis of the daily headache activity of patient SE revealed that headache levels were highest on Mondays and Thursdays and lowest on weekends. Although a great variety of situations was capable of triggering a tension headache; e.g. forgetting a shopping list, losing the car keys or preparing dinner for company, the most frequent cause was meeting with her supervisor in the early afternoon. It is interesting to note that 2.00 p.m. was, on the average, the hour of greatest headache activity.

Patient SE first noticed a decline in headache during the third week of training; however, analysis of the daily headache data revealed a gradual decline beginning with the first week of training. In all, this patient received 9 weeks of training during which she showed declining EMG and headache activity levels (see Fig. 2 which shows headache levels for baseline period and the *first 4* weeks of feedback training).

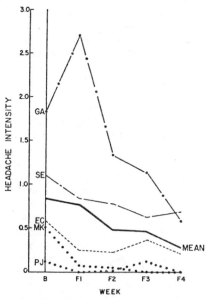

FIG. 2. Tension headache levels for each of five patients over a 5 week period.

Another important feature of the training process—and one which is significant in this type of procedure—is that the patient acquired some ability to produce the relaxation response outside the laboratory. Since many of the headaches occurred in the early afternoon she was encouraged to practise relaxing in her office during the lunch hour. She attempted to relax in her chair for a period of from 10 to 20 min.

A follow-up interview, 3 months after termination of training showed that tension headaches had virtually disappeared and that the patient was in good spirits generally. There was no evidence of symptom substitution.

Patient 2

MK was a middle-aged housewife who had suffered from frequent tension headaches over the previous 3 years. With feedback training she learned to relax rather quickly and was subsequently shifted from the lying to the sitting position for her last training sessions. This patient received training over an 11-week period. As can be seen in Fig. 2, headache activity showed a substantial decrease even in the first week of training.

Whereas MK had originally shown a tendency to overreact to minor stresses, she reported after training that such lesser events, over which she had little or no control, no longer upset her.

The 3-month follow-up revealed an all but complete elimination of tension headaches.

Patient 3

The third patient (EC) was a young high school teacher married to a medical student. She had been afflicted with tension headaches ever since graduating from college 2 years previously. Because the patient had to leave town with her husband within 5 weeks she was seen three times a week. As may be seen in Fig. 2 her headache activity dropped off rapidly, and remained low throughout the training period; but, after she left the area, increased again. This increase was due to the fact that she was beginning a new teaching job and, in the crush of new duties, had neglected to take time out to relax each day. She was advised to reinstate the daily relaxation period. The headache activity subsequently decreased again to the low levels attained during the training periods and has remained there for the duration of the 3-month post-training period.

Patient 4

Although PJ, a 33-year-old housewife, had reported a moderate level of headache activity over a period of 3 years, her baseline period showed only low headache activity. However, she continued in the program and learned very quickly to produce low frontalis EMG levels. Her headache activity remained low during training, a period of 3 months. Moreover, she reported that she was sleeping more soundly than before and was less likely to awaken from slight noises during the night—an observation consistent with the reports of Jacobson (1938) and Schultz and Luthe (1959) that training in deep muscle relaxation is frequently useful in treating sleep-onset insomnia.

A 2-month follow-up revealed that headache activity had remained at low levels.

Patient 5

Patient GA was a dynamic, middle-aged businessman who, ever since early adolescence, had suffered from frequent and severe tension headaches. He had previously received some training in deep relaxation while undergoing behavior therapy. Consequently, he learned to relax his frontalis muscle very quickly and was able to maintain low EMG levels at all times during feedback training. Although his baseline headache activity was very high, it decreased rapidly during the second week of training and remained low for the duration of the training.

After his fourth week of feedback training, the patient went on a 5-week vacation. Upon his return to work his headaches also returned. Significantly, the patient had neglected his daily relaxation session. He reported he had to "get things back in order" after his vacation, and was in a state of high tension. He was then given two more feedback sessions and was strongly

advised to schedule a period of relaxation practice every day. His headache activity then returned to low levels and has remained there for the rest of the 3-month post-training period.

COMBINED RESULTS

The data from the daily headache charts were analyzed so that each patient's headache activity was specified as an hourly average for each week of the experiment. Data from all five subjects were averaged to produce the graphs in Fig. 3. Both headache activity and frontalis EMG levels (weekly means) showed declines as training progressed.

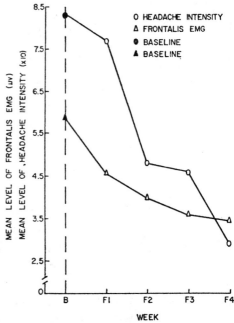

FIG. 3. Mean tension headache levels and mean frontalis EMG levels for five patients over a 5-week period.

A sign test (Siegel, 1956) showed that there was a significant difference ($P < 0.03$ one-tailed) between headache activity during the baseline period and the average for the third and fourth weeks of feedback training. This same test revealed a significant difference ($P < 0.03$) between baseline EMG levels and an average of the levels for the third and fourth weeks.

It should be noted that Figs. 2 and 3 illustrate results for a baseline period and 4 training weeks even though four of the five patients received training for longer periods of time. Patient GA began a 5-week vacation at the end of the fourth week of training. The remaining four patients continued to show decreasing headache and frontalis EMG activity in the additional training weeks.

As the patients progressed through the program they reported that changes were taking place in their day-to-day lives outside the laboratory environment. These changes were characterized by:

(1) A heightened awareness of maladaptive rising tension.

(2) An increasing ability to reduce such tension.

(3) A decreasing tendency to overreact to stress, e.g. "Things don't seem to bother me as much as they used to".

The first two changes were most probably directly related to the EMG bio-feedback training in the laboratory. The third change was perhaps due to a general lowering of arousal level as a result of the daily relaxation periods outside the laboratory.

DISCUSSION

Although this pilot study involves only a small number of cases and does not employ control groups, it is of interest for several reasons: (1) A novel technique, and one directly relevant to modifying or eliminating the presumed immediate cause of muscle contraction or tension headache, was successfully applied to the treatment of five patients suffering from the disorder. Diminution of headache activity was closely time-locked with the onset of the EMG-feedback training. Follow-up results over a 3-month period indicates that headache activity remains at a low level especially if patients continue relaxing for a short time each day. (2) In view of the high incidence of tension headache in the general population, the method of treatment outlined in this paper should have considerable practical significance. (3) The daily headache charts introduced in this study proved to be very useful for purposes of data analysis—both as a means of quantifying headache activity and as a way of determining the situations likely to trigger a headache. As the patients charted daily headache activity they became more aware of the specific precipitating stresses. (4) After their bio-feedback training, the patients seemed more able to exclude tension-evoking thoughts. Such an ability is useful because success in relaxing striate musculature seems to be partly determined by the individual's skill to exclude worrisome thoughts. (5) After a period of training the patients found that by relaxing they were able to decrease headache incidence and to abort slight-to-moderate intensity headaches. They became more aware of rising muscle tension, especially in the head and neck area, and were able to relax these muscles even if they were not lying down.

In general, the results of this pilot study seem to indicate that chronic tension headache sufferers can be trained to voluntarily lower their striate muscle tension in the face of daily life stresses and to reduce the incidence of tension headaches. Training does not use the usual psychotherapy methods or any drugs. The duration of the training period to achieve effective results appears to be 4–8 weeks.

The bio-feedback relaxation technique seems to be applicable to a number of psychosomatic and anxiety disorders. Indeed, pilot work in our laboratory suggests that EMG-feedback can be fruitfully combined with the behavior therapy technique of desensitization (Wolpe, 1958), and can be used to help relaxation training and the process of desensitizing the patient to anxiety-evoking thoughts.

Viewed in a broader context, the training of the muscle relaxation response described in this paper suggests that operant conditioning techniques may be successfully applied to certain events within the skin of the organism as well as to externally visible responses. Perhaps such application to private events may develop into a major new point of departure for operant techniques. If human subjects can be taught greater mastery over their internal environment, then the practical applications are considerable. In this study the feedback technique was applied simply to muscle activity. But in the light of Miller's work (1969) on the operant conditioning of a variety of autonomic responses in animals, the use of information feedback techniques in teaching control of certain autonomic responses in humans would also seem to be well worth exploring.

The possibilities of extending the range of operant methods by means of the information feedback technique has been discussed at greater length by Stoyva and Kamiya (1968) and Stoyva (1970). As described in these papers, the information feedback technique embodies a synthesis of elements from electronics, psychophysiology and operant conditioning. The core of the technique—precise measurement and amplification of a particular response, information feedback, and 'shaping'—would seem potentially applicable to a variety of physiological events.

REFERENCES

BUDZYNSKI T. H. and STOYVA J. M. (1969) An instrument for producing deep muscle relaxation by means of analog information feedback, *J. appl. Behav. Anal.* **2**, 231–237.

JACOBSON E. (1938) *Progressive Relaxation.* University of Chicago, Chicago.

MARTIN M. J. (1966) Tension headache, a psychiatric study, *Headache* **6**, 47–54.

MILLER N. E. (1969) Learning of visceral and glandular responses. *Science* **163**, 434–445.

OSTFELD A. M. (1962) *The Common Headache Syndromes: Biochemistry, Pathophysiology, Therapy.* Thomas, Springfield, Illinois.

SCHULTZ J. H. and LUTHE W. (1959) *Autogenic Training: A Psychophysiologic Approach in Psychotherapy.* Grune and Stratton, New York.

SHAW J. C. (1967) Integration technique. In *Manual of Psycho-Physiological Methods.* (Eds.: P. H. Venables and I. Martin), pp. 403–465. Wiley, New York.

SIEGEL S. (1956) *Nonparametric Statistics*, p. 75. McGraw-Hill, New York.

STOYVA J. M. and KAMIYA J. (1968) Electrophysiological studies of dreaming as the prototype of a new strategy in the study of consciousness, *Psychol. Rev.* **75**, 192–205.

STOYVA J. M. (1970) The public (scientific) study of private events. In *Sleep and Dreaming.* (Ed. E. Hartmann.) pp. 355–368, Little-Brown, Boston.

WOLFF H. G. (1963) *Headache and Other Head Pain.* Oxford University Press, New York.

WOLPE J. (1958) *Psychotherapy by Reciprocal Inhibition.* Stanford University Press, Stanford, California.

Learning of Visceral and Glandular Responses

Neal E. Miller

There is a strong traditional belief in the inferiority of the autonomic nervous system and the visceral responses that it controls. The recent experiments disproving this belief have deep implications for theories of learning, for individual differences in autonomic responses, for the cause and the cure of abnormal psychosomatic symptoms, and possibly also for the understanding of normal homeostasis. Their success encourages investigators to try other unconventional types of training. Before describing these experiments, let me briefly sketch some elements in the history of the deeply entrenched, false belief in the gross inferiority of one major part of the nervous system.

Historical Roots and

Modern Ramifications

Since ancient times, reason and the voluntary responses of the skeletal muscles have been considered to be superior, while emotions and the presumably involuntary glandular and visceral responses have been considered to be inferior. This invidious dichotomy appears in the philosophy of Plato (1), with his superior rational soul in the

SCIENCE, 1969, vol. 163, pp. 434-445.

head above and inferior souls in the body below. Much later, the great French neuroanatomist Bichat (2) distinguished between the cerebrospinal nervous system of the great brain and spinal cord, controlling skeletal responses, and the dual chain of ganglia (which he called "little brains") running down on either side of the spinal cord in the body below and controlling emotional and visceral responses. He indicated his low opinion of the ganglionic system by calling it "vegetative"; he also believed it to be largely independent of the cerebrospinal system, an opinion which is still reflected in our modern name for it, the autonomic nervous system. Considerably later, Cannon (3) studied the sympathetic part of the autonomic nervous system and concluded that the different nerves in it all fire simultaneously and are incapable of the finely differentiated individual responses possible for the cerebrospinal system, a conclusion which is enshrined in modern textbooks.

Many, though not all, psychiatrists have made an invidious distinction between the hysterical and other symptoms that are mediated by the cerebrospinal nervous system and the psychosomatic symptoms that are mediated by the autonomic nervous system. Whereas the former are supposed to be subject to a higher type of control that is symbolic, the latter are presumed to be only the direct physiological consequences of the type and intensity of the patient's emotions (see, for example, 4).

Similarly, students of learning have made a distinction between a lower form, called classical conditioning and thought to be involuntary, and a superior form variously called trial-and-error learning, operant conditioning, type II conditioning, or instrumental learning and believed to be responsible for voluntary behavior. In classical conditioning, the reinforcement must be by an unconditioned stimulus that already elicits the specific response to be learned; therefore, the possibilities are quite limited. In instrumental learning, the reinforcement, called a reward, has the property of strengthening any immediately preceding response. Therefore, the possibilities for reinforcement are much greater; a given reward may reinforce any one of a number of different responses, and a given response may be reinforced by any one of a number of different rewards.

Finally, the foregoing invidious distinctions have coalesced into the strong traditional belief that the superior type of instrumental learning involved in the superior voluntary behavior is possible only for skeletal responses mediated by the superior cerebrospinal nervous system, while, conversely, the inferior classical conditioning is the only kind possible for the inferior, presumably involuntary, visceral and emotional responses mediated by the inferior autonomic nervous system. Thus, in a recent summary generally considered authoritative, Kimble (5) states the almost universal belief that "for autonomically mediated behavior, the evidence points unequivocally to the conclusion that such responses can be modified by classical, but not instrumental, training methods." Upon examining the evidence, however, one finds that it consists only of failure to secure instrumental learning in two incompletely reported exploratory experiments and a vague allusion to the Russian literature (6). It is only against a cultural background of great prejudice that such weak evidence could lead to such a strong conviction.

The belief that instrumental learning is possible only for the cerebrospinal system and, conversely, that the autonomic nervous system can be modified only by classical conditioning has been used as one of the strongest arguments for the notion that instrumental learning and classical conditioning are two basically different phenomena rather than different manifestations of the same phenomenon under different conditions. But for many years I have been impressed with the similarity between the laws of classical conditioning and those of instrumental learning, and with the fact that, in each of these two situations, some of the specific details of learning vary with the specific conditions of learning. Failing to see any clear-cut dichotomy, I have assumed that there is only one kind of learning (7). This assumption has logically demanded that instrumental training procedures be able to produce the learning of any visceral responses that could be acquired through classical conditioning procedures. Yet it was only a little over a dozen years ago that I began some experimental work on this problem and a somewhat shorter time ago that I first, in published articles (8), made specific sharp challenges to the traditional view that the instrumental learning of visceral responses is impossible.

Some Difficulties

One of the difficulties of investigating

the instrumental learning of visceral responses stems from the fact that the responses that are the easiest to measure —namely, heart rate, vasomotor responses, and the galvanic skin response —are known to be affected by skeletal responses, such as exercise, breathing, and even tensing of certain muscles, such as those in the diaphragm. Thus, it is hard to rule out the possibility that, instead of directly learning a visceral response, the subject has learned a skeletal response the performance of which causes the visceral change being recorded.

One of the controls I planned to use was the paralysis of all skeletal responses through administration of curare, a drug which selectively blocks the motor end plates of skeletal muscles without eliminating consciousness in human subjects or the neural control of visceral responses, such as the beating of the heart. The muscles involved in breathing are paralyzed, so the subject's breathing must be maintained through artificial respiration. Since it seemed unlikely that curarization and other rigorous control techniques would be easy to use with human subjects, I decided to concentrate first on experiments with animals.

Originally I thought that learning would be more difficult when the animal was paralyzed, under the influence of curare, and therefore I decided to postpone such experiments until ones on nonparalyzed animals had yielded some definitely promising results. This turned out to be a mistake because, as I found out much later, paralyzing the animal with curare not only greatly simplifies the problem of recording visceral responses without artifacts introduced by movement but also apparently makes it easier for the animal to learn, perhaps because paralysis of the skeletal muscles removes sources of variability and distraction. Also, in certain experiments I made the mistake of using rewards that induced

strong unconditioned responses that interfered with instrumental learning.

One of the greatest difficulties, however, was the strength of the belief that instrumental learning of glandular and visceral responses is impossible. It was extremely difficult to get students to work on this problem, and when paid assistants were assigned to it, their attempts were so half-hearted that it soon became more economical to let them work on some other problem which they could attack with greater faith and enthusiasm. These difficulties and a few preliminary encouraging but inconclusive early results have been described elsewhere (9).

Success with Salivation

The first clear-cut results were secured by Alfredo Carmona and me in an experiment on the salivation of dogs. Initial attempts to use food as a reward for hungry dogs were unsuccessful, partly because of strong and persistent unconditioned salivation elicited by the food. Therefore, we decided to use water as a reward for thirsty dogs. Preliminary observations showed that the water had no appreciable effects one way or the other on the bursts of spontaneous salivation. As an additional precaution, however, we used the experimental design of rewarding dogs in one group whenever they showed a burst of spontaneous salivation, so that they would be trained to increase salivation, and rewarding dogs in another group whenever there was a long interval between spontaneous bursts, so that they would be trained to decrease salivation. If the reward had any unconditioned effect, this effect might be classically conditioned to the experimental situation and therefore produce a change in salivation that was not a true instance of instrumental learning. But in classical conditioning the reinforcement must

116

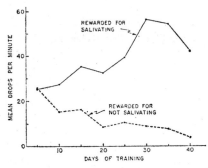

Fig. 1. Learning curves for groups of thirsty dogs rewarded with water for either increases or decreases in spontaneous salivation. [From Miller and Carmona (10)]

elicit the response that is to be acquired. Therefore, conditioning of a response elicited by the reward could produce either an increase or a decrease in salivation, depending upon the direction of the unconditioned response elicited by the reward, but it could not produce a change in one direction for one group and in the opposite direction for the other group. The same type of logic applies for any unlearned cumulative aftereffects of the reward; they could not be in opposite directions for the two groups. With instrumental learning, however, the reward can reinforce any response that immediately precedes it; therefore, the same reward can be used to produce either increases or decreases.

The results are presented in Fig. 1, which summarizes the effects of 40 days of training with one 45-minute training session per day. It may be seen that in this experiment the learning proceeded slowly. However, statistical analysis showed that each of the trends in the predicted rewarded direction was highly reliable (10).

Since the changes in salivation for the two groups were in opposite directions, they cannot be attributed to classical conditioning. It was noted, however, that the group rewarded for increases seemed to be more aroused and active than the one rewarded for decreases.

Conceivably, all we were doing was to change the level of activation of the dogs, and this change was, in turn, affecting the salivation. Although we did not observe any specific skeletal responses, such as chewing movements or panting, which might be expected to elicit salivation, it was difficult to be absolutely certain that such movements did not occur. Therefore, we decided to rule out such movements by paralyzing the dogs with curare, but we immediately found that curare had two effects which were diastrous for this experiment: it elicited such copious and continuous salivation that there were no changes in salivation to reward, and the salivation was so viscous that it almost immediately gummed up the recording apparatus.

Heart Rate

In the meantime, Jay Trowill, working with me on this problem, was displaying great ingenuity, courage, and persistence in trying to produce instrumental learning of heart rate in rats that had been paralyzed by curare to prevent them from "cheating" by muscular exertion to speed up the heart or by relaxation to slow it down. As a result of preliminary testing, he selected a dose of curare (3.6 milligrams of d-tubocurarine chloride per kilogram, injected intraperitoneally) which produced deep paralysis for at least 3 hours, and a rate of artificial respiration (inspiration-expiration ratio 1:1; 70 breaths per minute; peak pressure reading, 20 cm-H_2O) which maintained the heart at a constant and normal rate throughout this time.

In subsequent experiments, DiCara and I have obtained similar effects by starting with a smaller dose (1.2 milligrams per kilogram) and constantly infusing additional amounts of the drug, through intraperitoneal injection, at the rate of 1.2 milligrams per kilogram per hour, for the duration of the experiment. We have recorded, electromyographically, the response of the muscles, to determine that this dose does indeed produce a complete block of the action potentials, lasting for at least an hour after the end of infusion. We have found that if parameters of respiration and the face mask are adjusted carefully, the procedure not only maintains the heart rate of a 500-gram control animal constant but also maintains the vital signs of temperature, peripheral vasomotor responses, and the pCO_2 of the blood constant.

Since there are not very many ways to reward an animal completely paralyzed by curare, Trowill and I decided to use direct electrical stimulation of rewarding areas of the brain. There were other technical difficulties to overcome, such as devising the automatic system for rewarding small changes in heart rate as recorded by the electrocardiogram. Nevertheless, Trowill at last succeeded in training his rats (11). Those rewarded for an increase in heart rate showed a statistically reliable increase, and those rewarded for a decrease in heart rate showed a statistically reliable decrease. The changes, however, were disappointingly small, averaging only 5 percent in each direction.

The next question was whether larger changes could be achieved by improving the technique of training. DiCara and I used the technique of shaping—in other words, of immediately rewarding first very small, and hence frequently occurring, changes in the correct direction and, as soon as these had been learned, requiring progressively larger changes as the criterion for reward. In this way, we were able to produce in 90 minutes of training changes averaging 20 percent in either direction (12).

Key Properties of Learning: Discrimination and Retention

Does the learning of visceral responses have the same properties as the learning of skeletal responses? One of the important characteristics of the instrumental learning of skeletal responses is that a discrimination can be learned, so that the responses are more likely to be made in the stimulus situations in which they are rewarded than in those in which they are not. After the training of the first few rats had convinced us that we could produce large changes in heart rate, DiCara and I gave all the rest of the rats in the experiment described above 45 minutes of additional training with the most difficult criterion. We did this in order to see whether they could learn to give a greater response during a "time-in" stimulus (the presence of a flashing light and a tone) which indicated that a response in the proper direction would be rewarded than during a "time-out" stimulus (absence of light and tone) which indicated that a correct response would not be rewarded.

Figure 2 shows the record of one of the rats given such training. Before the beginning of the special discrimination training it had slowed its heart from an initial rate of 350 beats per minute to a rate of 230 beats per minute. From the top record of Fig. 2 one can see that, at the beginning of the special discrimination training, there was no appreciable reduction in heart rate that was specifically associated with the time-in stimulus. Thus it took the rat considerable time after the onset of this stimulus to meet the criterion and get the reward. At the end of the discrimination training the heart rate during time-out remained approximately the same, but when the time-in light and tone came on, the heart slowed down and the criterion was promptly met. Although the other rats showed less

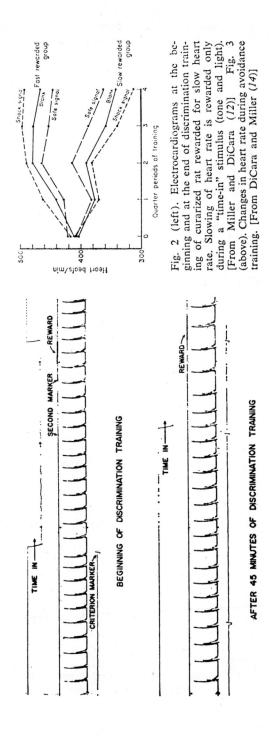

Fig. 2 (left). Electrocardiograms at the beginning and at the end of discrimination training of curarized rat rewarded for slow heart rate. Slowing of heart rate is rewarded only during a "time-in" stimulus (tone and light). [From Miller and DiCara (12)] Fig. 3 (above). Changes in heart rate during avoidance training. [From DiCara and Miller (14)]

change than this, by the end of the relatively short period of discrimination training their heart rate did change reliably ($P < .001$) in the predicted direction when the time-in stimulus came on. Thus, it is clear that instrumental visceral learning has at least one of the important properties of instrumental skeletal learning—namely, the ability to be brought under the control of a discriminative stimulus.

Another of the important properties of the instrumental learning of skeletal responses is that it is remembered. DiCara and I performed a special experiment to test the retention of learned changes in heart rate (13). Rats that had been given a single training session were returned to their home cages for 3 months without further training. When curarized again and returned to the experimental situation for nonreinforced test trials, rats in both the "increase" and the "decrease" groups showed good retention by exhibiting reliable changes in the direction rewarded in the earlier training.

Escape and Avoidance Learning

Is visceral learning by any chance peculiarly limited to reinforcement by the unusual reward of direct electrical stimulation of the brain, or can it be reinforced by other rewards in the same way that skeletal learning can be? In order to answer this question, DiCara and I (14) performed an experiment using the other of the two forms of thoroughly studied reward that can be conveniently used with rats which are paralyzed by curare—namely, the chance to avoid, or escape from, mild electric shock. A shock signal was turned on; after it had been on for 10 seconds it was accompanied by brief pulses of mild electric shock delivered to the rat's tail. During the first 10 seconds the rat could turn off the shock signal and avoid the shock by making the correct response of changing its heart rate in the required direction by the required amount. If it did not make the correct response in time, the shocks continued to be delivered until the rat escaped them by making the correct response, which immediately turned off both the shock and the shock signal.

For one group of curarized rats, the correct response was an increase in heart rate; for the other group it was a decrease. After the rats had learned to make small responses in the proper direction, they were required to make larger ones. During this training the shock signals were randomly interspersed with an equal number of "safe" signals that were not followed by shock; the heart rate was also recorded during so-called blank trials—trials without any signals or shocks. For half of the rats the shock signal was a tone and the "safe" signal was a flashing light; for the other half the roles of these cues were reversed.

The results are shown in Fig. 3. Each of the 12 rats in this experiment changed its heart rate in the rewarded direction. As training progressed, the shock signal began to elicit a progressively greater change in the rewarded direction than the change recorded during the blank trials; this was a statistically reliable trend. Conversely, as training progressed, the "safe" signal came to elicit a statistically reliable change in the opposite direction, toward the initial base line. These results show learning when escape and avoidance are the rewards; this means that visceral responses in curarized rats can be reinforced by rewards other than direct electrical stimulation of the brain. These rats also discriminate between the shock and the "safe" signals. You will remember that, with noncurarized thirsty dogs, we were able to use yet another kind of reward, water, to produce learned changes in salivation.

Transfer to Noncurarized State: More Evidence against Mediation

In the experiments discussed above, paralysis of the skeletal muscles by curare ruled out the possibility that the subjects were learning the overt performance of skeletal responses which were indirectly eliciting the changes in the heart rate. It is barely conceivable, however, that the rats were learning to send out from the motor cortex central impulses which would have activated the muscles had they not been paralyzed. And it is barely conceivable that these central impulses affected heart rate by means either of inborn connections or of classically conditioned ones that had been acquired when previous exercise had been accompanied by an increase in heart rate and relaxation had been accompanied by a decrease. But, if the changes in heart rate were produced in this indirect way, we would expect that, during a subsequent test without curare, any rat that showed learned changes in heart rate would show the movements in the muscles that were no longer paralyzed. Furthermore, the problem of whether or not visceral responses learned under curarization carry over to the noncurarized state is of interest in its own right.

In order to answer this question, Di-Cara and I (15) trained two groups of curarized rats to increase or decrease, respectively, their heart rate in order to avoid, or escape from, brief pulses of mild electric shock. When these rats were tested 2 weeks later in the noncurarized state, the habit was remembered. Statistically reliable increases in heart rate averaging 5 percent and decreases averaging 16 percent occurred. Immediately subsequent retraining without curare produced additional significant changes of heart rate in the rewarded direction, bringing the total overall increase to 11 percent and the decrease to 22 percent. While, at the beginning of the test in the noncurarized state, the two groups showed some differences in respiration and activity, these differences decreased until, by the end of the retraining, they were small and far from statistically reliable ($t = 0.3$ and 1.3, respectively). At the same time, the difference between the two groups with respect to heart rate was increasing, until it became large and thus extremely reliable ($t = 8.6$, d.f. = 12, $P < .001$).

In short, while greater changes in heart rate were being learned, the response was becoming more specific, involving smaller changes in respiration and muscular activity. This increase in specificity with additional training is another point of similarity with the instrumental learning of skeletal responses. Early in skeletal learning, the rewarded correct response is likely to be accompanied by many unnecessary movements. With additional training during which extraneous movements are not rewarded, they tend to drop out.

It is difficult to reconcile the foregoing results with the hypothesis that the differences in heart rate were mediated primarily by a difference in either respiration or amount of general activity. This is especially true in view of the research, summarized by Ehrlich and Malmo (16), which shows that muscular activity, to affect heart rate in the rat, must be rather vigorous.

While it is difficult to rule out completely the possibility that changes in heart rate are mediated by central impulses to skeletal muscles, the possibility of such mediation is much less attractive for other responses, such as intestinal contractions and the formation of urine by the kidney. Furthermore, if the learning of these different responses can be shown to be specific in enough visceral responses, one runs out of different skeletal movements each eliciting a specific different visceral response

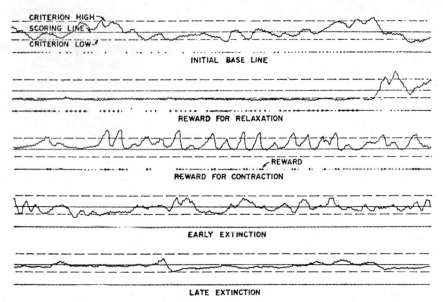

CRITERION HIGH
SCORING LINE
CRITERION LOW

INITIAL BASE LINE

REWARD FOR RELAXATION

REWARD
REWARD FOR CONTRACTION

EARLY EXTINCTION

LATE EXTINCTION

Fig. 4. Typical samples of a record of instrumental learning of an intestinal response by a curarized rat. (From top to bottom) Record of spontaneous contraction before training; record after training with reward for relaxation; record after training with reward for contractions; records during nonrewarded extinction trials. [From Miller and Banuazizi (*18*)]

(*17*). Therefore, experiments were performed on the learning of a variety of different visceral responses and on the specificity of that learning. Each of these experiments was, of course, interesting in its own right, quite apart from any bearing on the problem of mediation.

Specificity: Intestinal versus Cardiac

The purpose of our next experiment was to determine the specificity of visceral learning. If such learning has the same properties as the instrumental learning of skeletal responses, it should be possible to learn a specific visceral response independently of other ones. Furthermore, as we have just seen, we might expect to find that, the better the rewarded response is learned, the more specific is the learning. Banuazizi and I

worked on this problem (*18*). First we had to discover another visceral response that could be conveniently recorded and rewarded. We decided on intestinal contractions, and recorded them in the curarized rat with a little balloon filled with water thrust approximately 4 centimeters beyond the anal sphincter. Changes of pressure in the balloon were transduced into electric voltages which produced a record on a polygraph and also activated an automatic mechanism for delivering the reward, which was electrical stimulation of the brain.

The results for the first rat trained, which was a typical one, are shown in Fig. 4. From the top record it may be seen that, during habituation, there were some spontaneous contractions. When the rat was rewarded by brain stimulation for keeping contractions below a certain amplitude for a certain time, the number of contractions was reduced and the base line was lowered. After the record showed a highly reliable change indicating that relaxation had been learned (Fig. 4, second record from the top), the conditions of training were reversed and the reward was delivered whenever the amplitude of contractions rose above a certain level. From the next record (Fig. 4, middle) it may be seen that this type of training increased the number of contractions and raised the base line. Finally (Fig. 4, two bottom records) the reward was discontinued and, as would be expected, the response continued for a while but gradually became extinguished, so that the activity eventually returned to approximately its original base-line level.

After studying a number of other rats in this way and convincing ourselves that the instrumental learning of intestinal responses was a possibility, we designed an experiment to test specificity. For all the rats of the experiment, both intestinal contractions and heart rate were recorded, but half the rats were rewarded for one of these responses and half were rewarded for the other response. Each of these two groups of rats was divided into two subgroups, rewarded, respectively, for increased and decreased response. The rats were completely paralyzed by curare, maintained on artificial respiration, and rewarded by electrical stimulation of the brain.

The results are shown in Figs. 5 and 6. In Fig. 5 it may be seen that the group rewarded for increases in intestinal contractions learned an increase, the group rewarded for decreases learned a decrease, but neither of these groups showed an appreciable change in heart rate. Conversely (Fig. 6), the group rewarded for increases in heart rate showed an increase, the group rewarded for decreases showed a decrease, but neither of these groups showed a

change in intestinal contractions.

The fact that each type of response changed when it was rewarded rules out the interpretation that the failure to secure a change when that change was not rewarded could have been due to either a strong and stable homeostatic regulation of that response or an inability of our techniques to measure changes reliably under the particular conditions of our experiment.

Each of the 12 rats in the experiment showed statistically reliable changes in the rewarded direction; for 11 the changes were reliable beyond the $P <$ .001 level, while for the 12th the changes were reliable only beyond the .05 level. A statistically reliable negative correlation showed that the better the rewarded visceral response was learned, the less change occurred in the other, nonrewarded response. This greater specificity with better learning is what we had expected. The results showed that visceral learning can be specific to an organ system, and they clearly ruled out the possibility of mediation by any single general factor, such as level of activation or central commands for either general activity or relaxation.

In an additional experiment, Banuazizi (19) showed that either increases or decreases in intestinal contractions can be rewarded by avoidance of, or escape from, mild electric shocks, and that the intestinal responses can be discriminatively elicited by a specific stimulus associated with reinforcement.

Kidney Function

Encouraged by these successes, DiCara and I decided to see whether or not the rate of urine formation by the kidney could be changed in the curarized rat rewarded by electrical stimulation of the brain (20). A catheter, permanently inserted, was used to prevent accumulation of urine by the bladder, and the rate of urine formation

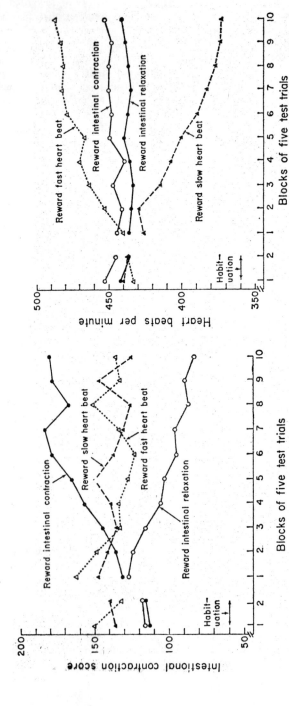

Fig. 5 (left). Graph showing that the intestinal contraction score is changed by rewarding either increases or decreases in intestinal contractions but is unaffected by rewarding changes in heart rate. [From Miller and Banuazizi (18)]   Fig. 6 (right). Graph showing that the heart rate is changed by rewarding either increases or decreases in heart rate but is unaffected by rewarding changes in intestinal contractions. Comparison with Fig. 5 demonstrates the specificity of visceral learning. [From Miller and Banuazizi (18)]

124

was measured by an electronic device for counting minute drops. In order to secure a rate of urine formation fast enough so that small changes could be promptly detected and rewarded, the rats were kept constantly loaded with water through infusion by way of a catheter permanently inserted in the jugular vein.

All of the seven rats rewarded when the intervals between times of urine-drop formation lengthened showed decreases in the rate of urine formation, and all of the seven rats rewarded when these intervals shortened showed increases in the rate of urine formation. For both groups the changes were highly reliable ($P < .001$).

In order to determine how the change in rate of urine formation was achieved, certain additional measures were taken. As the set of bars at left in Fig. 7 shows, the rate of filtration, measured by means of ^{14}C-labeled inulin, increased when increases in the rate of urine formation were rewarded and decreased when decreases in the rate were rewarded. Plots of the correlations showed that the changes in the rates of filtration and urine formation were not related to changes in either blood pressure or heart rate.

The middle set of bars in Fig. 7 shows that the rats rewarded for increases in the rate of urine formation had an increased rate of renal blood flow, as measured by ^{3}H-p-aminohippuric acid, and that those rewarded for decreases had a decreased rate of renal blood flow. Since these changes in blood flow were not accompanied by changes in general blood pressure or in heart rate, they must have been achieved by vasomotor changes of the renal arteries. That these vasomotor changes were at least somewhat specific is shown by the fact that vasomotor responses of the tail, as measured by a photoelectric plethysmograph, did not differ for the two groups of rats.

The set of bars at right in Fig. 7 shows that when decreases in rate of urine formation were rewarded, a more concentrated urine, having higher osmolarity, was formed. Since the slower passage of urine through the tubules

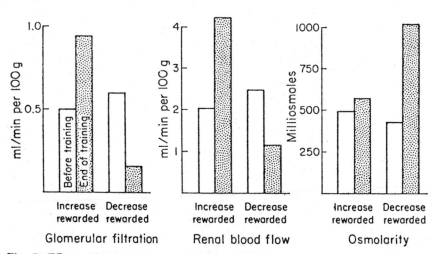

Fig. 7. Effects of rewarding increased rate of urine formation in one group and decreased rate in another on measures of glomerular filtration, renal blood flow, and osmolarity. [From data in Miller and DiCara (20)]

would afford more opportunity for re-absorption of water, this higher concentration does not necessarily mean an increase in the secretion of antidiuretic hormone. When an increased rate of urine formation was rewarded, the urine did not become more diluted—that is, it showed no decrease in osmolarity; therefore, the increase in rate of urine formation observed in this experiment cannot be accounted for in terms of an inhibition of the secretion of antidiuretic hormone.

From the foregoing results it appears that the learned changes in urine formation in this experiment were produced primarily by changes in the rate of filtration, which, in turn, were produced primarily by changes in the rate of blood flow through the kidneys.

Gastric Changes

In the next experiment, Carmona, Demierre, and I used a photoelectric plethysmograph to measure changes, presumably in the amount of blood, in the stomach wall (21). In an operation performed under anesthesia, a small glass tube, painted black except for a small spot, was inserted into the rat's stomach. The same tube was used to hold the stomach wall against a small glass window inserted through the body wall. The tube was left in that position. After the animal had recovered, a bundle of optical fibers could be slipped snugly into the glass tube so that the light beamed through it would shine out through the unpainted spot in the tube inside the stomach, pass through the stomach wall, and be recorded by a photocell on the other side of the glass window. Preliminary tests indicated that, as would be expected, when the amount of blood in the stomach wall increased, less light would pass through. Other tests showed that stomach contractions elicited by injections of insulin

did not affect the amount of light transmitted.

In the main experiment we rewarded curarized rats by enabling them to avoid or escape from mild electric shocks. Some were rewarded when the amount of light that passed through the stomach wall increased, while others were rewarded when the amount decreased. Fourteen of the 15 rats showed changes in the rewarded direction. Thus, we demonstrated that the stomach wall, under the control of the autonomic nervous system, can be modified by instrumental learning. There is strong reason to believe that the learned changes were achieved by vasomotor responses affecting the amount of blood in the stomach wall or mucosa, or in both.

In another experiment, Carmona (22) showed that stomach contractions can be either increased or decreased by instrumental learning.

It is obvious that learned changes in the blood supply of internal organs can affect their functioning—as, for example, the rate at which urine was formed by the kidneys was affected by changes in the amount of blood that flowed through them. Thus, such changes can produce psychosomatic symptoms. And if the learned changes in blood supply can be specific to a given organ, the symptom will occur in that organ rather than in another one.

Peripheral Vasomotor Responses

Having investigated the instrumental learning of internal vasomotor responses, we next studied the learning of peripheral ones. In the first experiment, the amount of blood in the tail of a curarized rat was measured by a photoelectric plethysmograph, and changes were rewarded by electrical stimulation of the brain (23). All of the four rats rewarded for vasoconstriction showed that response, and, at the same time, their average core temperature, measured rectally, decreased from 98.9° to 97.9°F. All of the four rats rewarded for vasodilatation showed that response and, at the same time, their average core temperature increased from 99.9° to 101°F. The vasomotor change for each individual rat was reliable beyond the $P < .01$ level, and the difference in change in temperature between the groups was reliable beyond the .01 level. The direction of the change in temperature was opposite to that which would be expected from the heat conservation caused by peripheral vasoconstriction or the heat loss caused by peripheral vasodilatation. The changes are in the direction which would be expected if the training had altered the rate of heat production, causing a change in temperature which, in turn, elicited the vasomotor response.

The next experiment was designed to try to determine the limits of the specificity of vasomotor learning. The pinnae of the rat's ears were chosen because the blood vessels in them are believed to be innervated primarily, and perhaps exclusively, by the sympathetic branch of the autonomic nervous system, the branch that Cannon believed always fired nonspecifically as a unit (3). But Cannon's experiments involved exposing cats to extremely strong emotion-evoking stimuli, such as barking dogs, and such stimuli will also evoke generalized activity throughout the skeletal musculature. Perhaps his results reflected the way in which sympathetic activity was elicited, rather than demonstrating any inherent inferiority of the sympathetic nervous system.

In order to test this interpretation, DiCara and I (24) put photocells on both ears of the curarized rat and connected them to a bridge circuit so that only differences in the vasomotor responses of the two ears were rewarded by brain stimulation. We were somewhat surprised and greatly delighted to find that this experiment actually worked. The results are summarized in Fig. 8. Each of the six rats rewarded for relative vasodilatation of the left ear showed that response, while each of the six rats rewarded for relative vasodilatation of the right ear showed that response. Recordings from the right and left forepaws showed little if any change in vasomotor response.

It is clear that these results cannot be by-products of changes in either heart rate or blood pressure, as these would be expected to affect both ears equally. They show either that vasomotor responses mediated by the sympathetic nervous system are capable of much greater specificity than has previously been believed, or that the innervation of the blood vessels in the pinnae of the ears is not restricted almost exclusively to sympathetic-nervous-system components, as has been believed, and involves functionally significant parasympathetic components. In any event, the changes in the blood flow certainly were surprisingly specific. Such changes in blood flow could account for specific psychosomatic symptoms.

Blood Pressure Independent of Heart Rate

Although changes in blood pressure were not induced as by-products of rewarded changes in the rate of urine formation, another experiment on curarized rats showed that, when changes in systolic blood pressure are specifically reinforced, they can be learned (25). Blood pressure was recorded by means of a catheter permanently inserted into the aorta, and the reward was avoidance of, or escape from, mild electric shock. All seven rats rewarded for increases in blood pressure showed further increases, while all seven rewarded for decreases showed decreases, each of the changes,

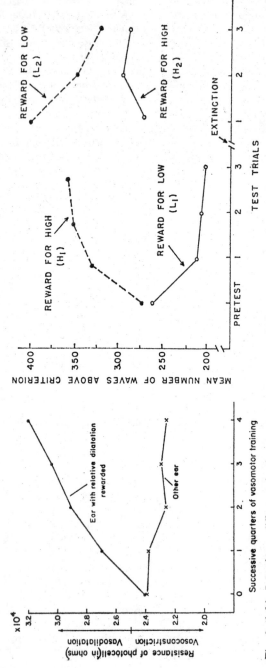

Fig. 8 (left). Learning a difference in the vasomotor responses of the two ears in the curarized rat. [From data in DiCara and Miller (24)]   Fig. 9 (right). Instrumental learning by curarized rats rewarded for high-voltage or for low-voltage electroencephalograms recorded from the cerebral cortex. After a period of nonrewarded extinction, which produced some drowsiness, as indicated by an increase in voltage, the rats in the two groups were then rewarded for voltage changes opposite in direction to the changes for which they were rewarded earlier. [From Carmona (29)]

128

which were in opposite directions, being reliable beyond the $P < .01$ level. The increase was from 139 mm-Hg, which happens to be roughly comparable to the normal systolic blood pressure of an adult man, to 170 mm-Hg, which is on the borderline of abnormally high blood pressure in man.

Each experimental animal was "yoked" with a curarized partner, maintained on artificial respiration and having shock electrodes on its tail wired in series with electrodes on the tail of the experimental animal, so that it received exactly the same electric shocks and could do nothing to escape or avoid them. The yoked controls for both the increase-rewarded and the decrease-rewarded groups showed some elevation in blood pressure as an unconditioned effect of the shocks. By the end of training, in contrast to the large difference in the blood pressures of the two groups specifically rewarded for changes in opposite directions, there was no difference in blood pressure between the yoked control partners for these two groups. Furthermore, the increase in blood pressure in these control groups was reliably less ($P < .01$) than that in the group specifically rewarded for increases. Thus, it is clear that the reward for an increase in blood pressure produced an additional increase over and above the effects of the shocks per se, while the reward for a decrease was able to overcome the unconditioned increase elicited by the shocks.

For none of the four groups was there a significant change in heart rate or in temperature during training; there were no significant differences in these measures among the groups. Thus, the learned change was relatively specific to blood pressure.

Transfer from Heart Rate
to Skeletal Avoidance

Although visceral learning can be quite specific, especially if only a specific response is rewarded, as was the case in the experiment on the two ears, under some circumstances it can involve a more generalized effect.

In handling the rats that had just recovered from curarization, DiCara noticed that those that had been trained, through the avoidance or escape reward, to increase their heart rate were more likely to squirm, squeal, defecate, and show other responses indicating emotionality than were those that had been trained to reduce their heart rate. Could instrumental learning of heart-rate changes have some generalized effects, perhaps on the level of emotionality, which might affect the behavior in a different avoidance-learning situation? In order to look for such an effect, DiCara and Weiss (26) used a modified shuttle avoidance apparatus. In this apparatus, when a danger signal is given, the rat must run from compartment A to compartment B. If he runs fast enough, he avoids the shock; if not, he must run to escape it. The next time the danger signal is given, the rat must run in the opposite direction, from B to A.

Other work had shown that learning in this apparatus is an inverted U-shaped function of the strength of the shocks, with shocks that are too strong eliciting emotional behavior instead of running. DiCara and Weiss trained their rats in this apparatus with a level of shock that is approximately optimum for naive rats of this strain. They found that the rats that had been rewarded for decreasing their heart rate learned well, but that those that had been rewarded for increasing their heart rate learned less well, as if their emotionality had been increased. The difference was statistically reliable ($P < .001$). This experiment clearly demonstrates that training a visceral response can affect the subsequent learning of a skeletal one, but additional work will be required to prove the hypothesis that training to increase heart rate increases emotionality.

Visceral Learning without Curare

Thus far, in all of the experiments except the one on teaching thirsty dogs to salivate, the initial training was given when the animal was under the influence of curare. All of the experiments, except the one on salivation, have produced surprisingly rapid learning—definitive results within 1 or 2 hours. Will learning in the normal, non-curarized state be easier, as we originally thought it should be, or will it be harder, as the experiment on the non-curarized dogs suggests? DiCara and I have started to get additional evidence on this problem. We have obtained clear-cut evidence that rewarding (with the avoidance or escape reward) one group of freely moving rats for reducing heart rate and rewarding another group for increasing heart rate produces a difference between the two groups (27). That this difference was not due to the indirect effects of the overt performance of skeletal responses is shown by the fact that it persisted in subsequent tests during which the rats were paralyzed by curare. And, on subsequent retraining without curare, such differences in activity and respiration as were present earlier in training continued to decrease, while the differences in heart rate continued to increase. It seems extremely unlikely that, at the end of training, the highly reliable differences in heart rate ($t = 7.2$; $P < .0001$) can be explained by the highly unreliable differences in activity and respiration ($t = .07$ and 0.2, respectively).

Although the rats in this experiment showed some learning when they were trained initially in the noncurarized state, this learning was much poorer than that which we have seen in our other experiments on curarized rats. This is exactly the opposite of my original expectation, but seems plausible in the light of hindsight. My hunch is that paralysis by curare improved learning by eliminating sources of distraction and variability. The stimulus situation was kept more constant, and confusing visceral fluctuations induced indirectly by skeletal movements were eliminated.

Learned Changes in Brain Waves

Encouraged by success in the experiments on the instrumental learning of visceral responses, my colleagues and I have attempted to produce other unconventional types of learning. Electrodes placed on the skull or, better yet, touching the surface of the brain record summative effects of electrical activity over a considerable area of the brain. Such electrical effects are called brain waves, and the record of them is called an electroencephalogram. When the animal is aroused, the electroencephalogram consists of fast, low-voltage activity; when the animal is drowsy or sleeping normally, the electroencephalogram consists of considerably slower, higher-voltage activity. Carmona attempted to see whether this type of brain activity, and the state of arousal accompanying it, can be modified by direct reward of changes in the brain activity (28, 29).

The subjects of the first experiment were freely moving cats. In order to have a reward that was under complete control and that did not require the cat to move, Carmona used direct electrical stimulation of the medial forebrain bundle, which is a rewarding area of the brain. Such stimulation produced a slight lowering in the average voltage of the electroencephalogram and an increase in behavioral arousal. In order to provide a control for these and any other unlearned effects, he rewarded one group for changes in the direction of high-voltage activity and another group for changes in the direction of low-voltage activity.

Both groups learned. The cats rewarded for high-voltage activity showed more high-voltage slow waves and tended to sit like sphinxes, staring out into space. The cats rewarded for low-voltage activity showed much more low-voltage fast activity, and appeared to be aroused, pacing restlessly about, sniffing, and looking here and there. It was clear that this type of training had modified both the character of the electrical brain waves and the general level of the behavioral activity. It was not clear, however, whether the level of arousal of the brain was directly modified and hence modified the behavior; whether the animals learned specific items of behavior which, in turn, modified the arousal of the brain as reflected in the electroencephalogram; or whether both types of learning were occurring simultaneously.

In order to rule out the direct sensory consequences of changes in muscular tension, movement, and posture, Carmona performed the next experiment on rats that had been paralyzed by means of curare. The results, given in Fig. 9, show that both rewarded groups showed changes in the rewarded direction; that a subsequent nonrewarded rest increased the number of high-voltage responses in both groups; and that, when the conditions of reward were reversed, the direction of change in voltage was reversed.

At present we are trying to use similar techniques to modify the functions of a specific part of the vagal nucleus, by recording and specifically rewarding changes in the electrical activity there. Preliminary results suggest that this is possible. The next step is to investigate the visceral consequences of such modification. This kind of work may open up possibilities for modifying the activity of specific parts of the brain and the functions that they control. In some cases, directly rewarding brain activity may be a more convenient or more powerful technique than rewarding skeletal or visceral behavior. It also may be a new way to throw light on the functions of specific parts of the brain (30).

Human Visceral Learning

Another question is that of whether people are capable of instrumental learning of visceral responses. I believe that in this respect they are as smart as rats. But, as a recent critical review by Katkin and Murray (31) points out, this has not yet been completely proved. These authors have comprehensively summarized the recent studies reporting successful use of instrumental training to modify human heart rate, vasomotor responses, and the galvanic skin response. Because of the difficulties in subjecting human subjects to the same rigorous controls, including deep paralysis by means of curare, that can be used with animal subjects, one of the most serious questions about the results of the human studies is whether the changes recorded represent the true instrumental learning of visceral responses or the unconscious learning of those skeletal responses that can produce visceral reactions. However, the able investigators who have courageously challenged the strong traditional belief in the inferiority of the autonomic nervous system with experiments at the more difficult but especially significant human level are developing ingenious controls, including demonstrations of the specificity of the visceral change, so that their cumulative results are becoming increasingly impressive.

Possible Role in Homeostasis

The functional utility of instrumental

learning by the cerebrospinal nervous system under the conditions that existed during mammalian evolution is obvious. The skeletal responses mediated by the cerebrospinal nervous system operate on the external environment, so that there is survival value in the ability to learn responses that bring rewards such as food, water, or escape from pain. The fact that the responses mediated by the autonomic nervous system do not have such direct action on the external environment was one of the reasons for believing that they are not subject to instrumental learning. Is the learning ability of the autonomic nervous system something that has no normal function other than that of providing my students with subject matter for publications? Is it a mere accidental by-product of the survival value of cerebrospinal learning, or does the instrumental learning of autonomically mediated responses have some adaptive function, such as helping to maintain that constancy of the internal environment called homeostasis?

In order for instrumental learning to function homeostatically, a deviation away from the optimum level will have to function as a drive to motivate learning, and a change toward the optimum level will have to function as a reward to reinforce the learning of the particular visceral response that produced the corrective change.

When a mammal has less than the optimum amount of water in his body, this deficiency serves as a drive of thirst to motivate learning; the overt consummatory response of drinking functions as a reward to reinforce the learning of the particular skeletal responses that were successful in securing the water that restored the optimum level. But is the consummatory response essential? Can restoration of an optimum level by a glandular response function as a reward?

In order to test for the possible rewarding effects of a glandular response, DiCara, Wolf, and I (32) injected albino rats with antidiuretic hormone (ADH) if they chose one arm of a T-maze and with the isotonic saline vehicle if they chose the other, distinctively different, arm. The ADH permitted water to be reabsorbed in the kidney, so that a smaller volume of more concentrated urine was formed. Thus, for normal rats loaded in advance with H_2O, the ADH interfered with the excess-water excretion required for the restoration of homeostasis, while the control injection of isotonic saline allowed the excess water to be excreted. And, indeed, such rats learned to select the side of the maze that assured them an injection of saline so that their glandular response could restore homeostasis.

Conversely, for rats with diabetes insipidus, loaded in advance with hypertonic NaCl, the homeostatic effects of the same two injections were reversed; the ADH, causing the urine to be more concentrated, helped the rats to get rid of the excess NaCl, while the isotonic saline vehicle did not. And, indeed, a group of rats of this kind learned the opposite choice of selecting the ADH side of the maze. As a further control on the effects of the ADH per se, normal rats which had not been given H_2O or NaCl exhibited no learning. This experiment showed that an excess of either H_2O or NaCl functions as a drive and that the return to the normal concentration produced by the appropriate response of a gland, the kidney, functions as a reward.

When we consider the results of this experiment together with those of our experiments showing that glandular and visceral responses can be instrumentally learned, we will expect the animal to learn those glandular and visceral responses mediated by the central nervous system that promptly restore homeostasis after any considerable deviation. Whether or not this theoretically possible learning has any practical significance will depend on whether or not the innate homeostatic mechanisms control the levels closely enough to prevent any deviations large enough to function as a drive from occurring. Even if the innate control should be accurate enough to preclude learning in most cases, there remains the intriguing possibility that, when pathology interferes with innate control, visceral learning is available as a supplementary mechanism.

Implications and Speculations

We have seen how the instrumental learning of visceral responses suggests a new possible homeostatic mechanism worthy of further investigation. Such learning also shows that the autonomic nervous system is not as inferior as has been so widely and firmly believed. It removes one of the strongest arguments for the hypothesis that there are two fundamentally different mechanisms of learning, involving different parts of the nervous system.

Cause of psychosomatic symptoms. Similarly, evidence of the instrumental learning of visceral responses removes the main basis for assuming that the psychosomatic symptoms that involve the autonomic nervous system are fundamentally different from those functional symptoms, such as hysterical ones, that involve the cerebrospinal nervous system. Such evidence allows us to extend to psychosomatic symptoms the type of learning-theory analysis that Dollard and I (7, 33) have applied to other symptoms.

For example, suppose a child is terror-stricken at the thought of going to school in the morning because he is completely unprepared for an important examination. The strong fear elicits a variety of fluctuating autonomic symptoms, such as a queasy stomach at one time and pallor and faintness at another; at this point his mother, who is partic-ularly concerned about cardiovascular symptoms, says, "You are sick and must stay home." The child feels a great relief from fear, and this reward should reinforce the cardiovascular responses producing pallor and faintness. If such experiences are repeated frequently enough, the child, theoretically, should learn to respond with that kind of symptom. Similarly, another child whose mother ignored the vasomotor responses but was particularly concerned by signs of gastric distress would learn the latter type of symptom. I want to exphasize, however, that we need careful clinical research to determine how frequently, if at all, the social conditions sufficient for such theoretically possible learning of visceral symptoms actually occur. Since a given instrumental response can be reinforced by a considerable variety of rewards, and by one reward on one occasion and a different reward on another, the fact that glandular and visceral responses can be instrumentally learned opens up many new theoretical possibilities for the reinforcement of psychosomatic symptoms.

Furthermore, we do not yet know how severe a psychosomatic effect can be produced by learning. While none of the 40 rats rewarded for speeding up their heart rates have died in the course of training under curarization, 7 of the 40 rats rewarded for slowing down their heart rates have died. This statistically reliable difference (chi square = 5.6, $P < .02$) is highly suggestive, but it could mean that training to speed up the heart helped the rats resist the stress of curare rather than that the reward for slowing down the heart was strong enough to overcome innate regulatory mechanisms and induce sudden death. In either event the visceral learning had a vital effect. At present, DiCara and I are trying to see whether or not the learning of visceral responses can be carried far enough in the noncurarized animal to produce physical damage. We are also investigating the possibility that there may be a critical period in early infancy during which visceral learning has particularly intense and long-lasting effects.

Individual and cultural differences. It is possible that, in addition to producing psychosomatic symptoms in extreme cases, visceral learning can account for certain more benign individual and cultural differences. Lacey and Lacey (*34*) have shown that a given individual may have a tendency, which is stable over a number of years, to respond to a variety of different stresses with the same profile of autonomic responses, while other individuals may have statistically reliable tendencies to respond with different profiles. It now seems possible that differential conditions of learning may account for at least some of these individual differences in patterns of autonomic response.

Conversely, such learning may account also for certain instances in which the same individual responds to the same stress in different ways. For example, a small boy who receives a severe bump in rough-and-tumble play may learn to inhibit the secretion of tears in this situation since his peer group will punish crying by calling it "sissy." But the same small boy may burst into tears when he gets home to his mother, who will not punish weeping and may even reward tears with sympathy.

Similarly, it seems conceivable that different conditions of reward by a culture different from our own may be responsible for the fact that Homer's adult heroes so often "let the big tears fall." Indeed, a former colleague of mine, Herbert Barry III, has analyzed cross-cultural data and found that the amount of crying reported for children seems to be related to the way in which the society reacts to their tears (*35*).

I have emphasized the possible role of learning in producing the observed individual differences in visceral responses to stress, which in extreme cases may result in one type of psychosomatic symptom in one person and a different type in another. Such learning does not, of course, exclude innate individual differences in the susceptibility of different organs. In fact, given social conditions under which any form of illness will be rewarded, the symptoms of the most susceptible organ will be the most likely ones to be learned. Furthermore, some types of stress may be so strong that the innate reactions to them produce damage without any learning. My colleagues and I are currently investigating the psychological variables involved in such types of stress (*36*).

Therapeutic training. The experimental work on animals has developed a powerful technique for using instrumental learning to modify glandular and visceral responses. The improved training technique consists of moment-to-moment recording of the visceral function and immediate reward, at first, of very small changes in the desired direction and then of progressively larger ones. The success of this technique suggests that it should be able to produce therapeutic changes. If the patient who is highly motivated to get rid of a symptom understands that a signal, such as a tone, indicates a change in the desired direction, that tone could serve as a powerful reward. Instruction to try to turn the tone on as often as possible and praise for success should increase the reward. As patients find that they can secure some control of the symptom, their motivation should be strengthened. Such a procedure should be well worth trying on any symptom, functional or organic, that is under neural control, that can be continuously monitored by modern instrumentation, and for which a given direction of change is clearly indicated medically— for example, cardiac arrhythmias, spastic colitis, asthma, and those cases of high blood pressure that are not essential compensation for kidney damage (37). The obvious cases to begin with are those in which drugs are ineffective or contraindicated. In the light of the fact that our animals learned so much better when under the influence of curare and transferred their training so well to the normal, nondrugged state, it should be worth while to try to use hypnotic suggestion to achieve similar results by enhancing the reward effect of the signal indicating a change in the desired direction, by producing relaxation and regular breathing, and by removing interference from skeletal responses and distraction by irrelevant cues.

Engel and Melmon (38) have reported encouraging results in the use of instrumental training to treat cardiac arrhythmias of organic origin. Randt, Korein, Carmona, and I have had some success in using the method described above to train epileptic patients in the laboratory to suppress, in one way or another, the abnormal paroxysmal spikes in their electroencephalogram. My colleagues and I are hoping to try learning therapy for other symptoms— for example, the rewarding of high-voltage electroencephalograms as a treatment for insomnia. While it is far too early to promise any cures, it certainly will be worth while to investigate thoroughly the therapeutic possibilities of improved instrumental training techniques.

References and Notes

1. *The Dialogues of Plato*, B. Jowett, Transl.. (Univ. of Oxford Press, London, ed. 2, 1875), vol. 3, "Timaeus."
2. X. Bichat, *Recherches Physiologiques sur la Vie et le Mort* (Brosson, Gabon, Paris, 1800).
3. W. B. Cannon, *The Wisdom of the Body* (Norton, New York, 1932).
4. F. Alexander, *Psychosomatic Medicine: Its Principles and Applications* (Norton, New York, 1950), pp. 40–41.
5. G. A. Kimble, *Hilgard and Marquis' Conditioning and Learning* (Appleton-Century-Crofts, New York, ed. 2, 1961), p. 100.
6. B. F. Skinner, *The Behavior of Organisms* (Appleton-Century, New York, 1938); O. H. Mowrer, *Harvard Educ. Rev.* 17, 102 (1947).
7. N. E. Miller and J. Dollard, *Social Learning and Imitation* (Yale Univ. Press, New Haven, 1941); J. Dollard and N. E. Miller, *Personality and Psychotherapy* (McGraw-Hill, New York, 1950); N. E. Miller, *Psychol. Rev.* 58, 375 (1951).
8. N. E. Miller, *Ann. N.Y. Acad. Sci.* 92, 830 (1961); ———, in *Nebraska Symposium on Motivation*, M. R. Jones, Ed. (Univ. of Nebraska Press, Lincoln, 1963); ———, in *Proc. 3rd World Congr. Psychiat., Montreal, 1961* (1963), vol. 3, p. 213.
9. ———, in "Proceedings, 18th International Congress of Psychology, Moscow, 1966," in press.
10. ——— and A. Carmona, *J. Comp. Physiol. Psychol.* 63, 1 (1967).
11. J. A. Trowill, ibid., p. 7.
12. N. E. Miller and L. V. DiCara, ibid., p. 12.
13. L. V. DiCara and N. E. Miller, *Commun. Behav. Biol.* 2, 19 (1968).
14. ———, *J. Comp. Physiol. Psychol.* 65, 8 (1968).
15. ———, ibid., in press.
16. D. J. Ehrlich and R. B. Malmo, *Neuropsychologia* 5, 219 (1967).
17. "It even becomes difficult to postulate enough different thoughts each arousing a different emotion, each of which in turn innately elicits a specific visceral response. And if one assumes a more direct specific connection between different thoughts and different visceral responses, the notion becomes indistinguishable from the ideo-motor hypothesis of the voluntary movement of skeletal muscles." [W. James, *Principles of Psychology* (Dover, New York, new ed., 1950), vol. 2, chap. 26].
18. N. E. Miller and A. Banuazizi, *J. Comp. Physiol. Psychol.* 65, 1 (1968).
19. A. Banuazizi, thesis, Yale University (1968).
20. N. E. Miller and L. V. DiCara, *Amer. J. Physiol.* 215, 677 (1968).
21. A. Carmona, N. E. Miller, T. Demierre, in preparation.
22. A. Carmona, in preparation.
23. L. V. DiCara and N. E. Miller, *Commun. Behav. Biol.* 1, 209 (1968).
24. ———, *Science* 159, 1485 (1968).
25. ———, *Psychosom. Med.* 30, 489 (1968).
26. L. V. DiCara and J. M. Weiss, *J. Comp. Physiol. Psychol.*, in press.
27. L. V. DiCara and N. E. Miller, *Physiol. Behav.*, in press.
28. N. E. Miller, *Science* 152, 676 (1966).
29. A. Carmona, thesis, Yale University (1967).
30. For somewhat similar work on the single-cell level, see J. Olds and M. E. Olds, in *Brain Mechanisms and Learning*, J. Delafresnaye, A. Fessard, J. Konorski, Eds. (Blackwell, London, 1961).
31. E. S. Katkin and N. E. Murray, *Psychol. Bull.* 70, 52 (1968); for a reply to their criticisms, see A. Crider, G. Schwartz, S. Shnidman, ibid., in press.
32. N. E. Miller, L. V. DiCara, G. Wolf, *Amer. J. Physiol.* 215, 684 (1968).
33. N. E. Miller, in *Personality Change*, D. Byrne and P. Worchel, Eds. (Wiley, New York, 1964), p. 149.
34. J. I. Lacey and B. C. Lacey, *Amer. J.*

Psychol. **71**, 50 (1958); *Ann. N.Y. Acad. Sci.* **98**, 1257 (1962).

35. H. Barry III, personal communication.
36. N. E. Miller, *Proc. N.Y. Acad. Sci.*, in press.
37. Objective recording of such symptoms might be useful also in monitoring the effects of quite different types of psychotherapy.
38. B. T. Engel and K. T. Melmon, personal communication.
39. The work described is supported by U.S. Public Health Service grant MH 13189.

DOES THE HEART LEARN?

DONALD SHEARN

In our time of cohabitation of various sciences one may wonder about the kind of affairs psychology has with some of the more firmly established disciplines. Other sciences may very well believe that the progeny of a relationship with psychology would necessarily be illegitimate. Or perhaps, at best, that psychology would have everything to gain and nothing to give. Must psychology be the protegee, or does it have unique techniques to share? It is the aim of this paper, by way of presenting some experimental findings, to suggest that certain techniques of modern psychology can be useful in the analysis of problems of cardiovascular physiology.

Detailed encouragement to the psychologist to use his techniques in the physiological laboratory comes from current adjustments in physiological thinking. Reviews of recent circulatory research by Rushmer (1955), Rushmer and Smith (1959), point out that the cardiovascular system is not altogether faithful to a few classical laws based largely upon simple hydraulic principles (Bainbridge, 1915; Patterson, Piper, & Starling, 1914). Rather it appears that this system is true to many principles roving about on several levels of analysis, among them the principles derived from conditioning procedures.

Gantt's translation of *The Internal Organs and the Cerebral Cortex* by Bykov (1957) could be the signal for a methodological revolution in certain phases of biological analysis and control, wherein the physiological reactions of the intact organism are modified by conditioning techniques. Of particular interest in this book for our present discussion is the chapter on circulatory adjustments. Several experiments are cited wherein cardiac, vasomotor, and even splenic responses are conditional upon exteroceptive stimuli presented by the experimenter.

In contrasting the results mentioned in the Bykov book with those from other sources we are brought to what is perhaps the most paradoxical feature of cardiovascular conditioning, the form of the conditioned cardiac response. Granting that the heart does learn, just what is it that is learned?

WHAT DOES THE HEART LEARN?

CR-UCR Similarity. Soviet investigators generally suggest that the conditioned response (CR) closely resembles the unconditioned response (UCR) as illustrated by an experiment of Petrova (Bykov, 1957). An auditory stimulus (whistle) was combined with intravenous injections of nitroglycerin. Because the act of injecting the fluid would act as a conditioned stimulus, its effect was extinguished with repeated intravenous injections of normal saline. The whistle, on the other hand, was always sounded after the nitroglycerin had been injected (but before the effect of the drug was manifest). After about 100 pairings of the whistle and nitroglycerin the whistle presented alone produced changes typical of those elicited by the drug (accelerated heart rate, decrease in QRS voltage, and augmented P and T waves). Delov (Bykov, 1957) demon-

PSYCHOLOGICAL BULLETIN, 1961, Vol. 58, pp. 452-458.

strated that a conditioned stimulus may produce a very different response from the above when combined a number of times with a drug of different consequences. In this experiment the conditioned stimulus (CS) was actually the stimulus complex associated with the injection, while the unconditioned stimulus (UCS) was a 0.2-gram injection of morphine. After 20 to 30 injections, the CS given without morphine produced the same changes in the electrocardiogram as those produced by morphine (deceleration in heart rate and marked reduction in the P deflection).

Additional experiments (Bykov, 1957) showing the similarity of UCR and CR for other drugs have been conducted by Samarin (strophanthin) and Levitin (acetylcholin and epinephrine).

Other investigators have taken a different view of the form of the heart rate CR. For example, in some experiments with human subjects by Zeaman, Deane, and Wegner (1954) and Zeaman and Wegner (1954), it was suggested that the CR resembles the UCR at the time of the UCS (shock) termination. In accord with this hypothesis a 2-second shock gave an accelerated heart rate CR and a 6-second shock gave a decelerated CR (since the UCR at shock termination was accelerating or decelerating, respectively). When other shock values were used in a later experiment (Zeaman & Wegner, 1958) this hypothesis was not upheld. It was predicted from the hypothesis that no conditioning would occur for a very short shock (0.1 second) which did not allow a change in heart rate before its termination, or for a very long shock (15 seconds) which allowed the heart rate to return to normal by the time it was termi-

nated. When conditioning did occur these investigators revised their hypothesis to suggest that to some extent large UCRs tend to give accelerative CRs and small UCRs decelerative CRs.

Decelerative CR. A decelerative heart rate CR in human subjects is consistently reported by Bersh, Notterman, and Schoenfeld (1953, 1956a, 1956b, 1956c, 1957a, 1957b; Notterman, Schoenfeld, & Bersh, 1952a, 1952b, 1952c). Their procedure was essentially the same as that used by Zeaman and Wegner (1954) with which a decelerative CR was obtained (1-second CS, 6-second CS-UCS interval, and a 6-second UCS). Their UCS shock level, however, was over twice that of the Zeaman and Wegner studies (30-volt alternating current as contrasted with 13-volt alternating current). For the most part, the measures indicating a decelerative CR were taken during the last two heart cycles of the CS-UCS interval. In answer to possible criticism that deceleration during this portion of the interval was not a representative CR, they also measured the first two heart cycles of the CS-UCS interval (Notterman et al., 1952c) and again found a decreasing heart rate, which was not, however, statistically significant.

Owens and Gantt (1950) report a decelerative CR when the petting of a dog served as the UCS. The UCR to this stimulation was also a reduction in heart rate. Mixed results regarding the form of the heart rate CR were obtained by Beier (1940). One subject showed an accelerative CR, another a decelerative CR, and still another, conditioned arrhythmia. The UCS used in this experiment was the working of a bicycle ergometer by the subject.

Accelerative CR. Other experiments

indicate a CR which is predominately accelerative in form. Skaggs (1926) used an auto horn CS and an induction shock UCS, separated by 1 minute, to produce a mild increase in human heart rate (1.1 beats/minute). A greater increase in rate was observed between the "normal" condition and the "expectancy" period preceding the CS (9.4 beats/minute).

Anderson and Parmenter (1941) demonstrated that the CR is an increase in heart rate when a buzzer or metronome CS is used with a shock pulse UCS. They further demonstrated "neurosis" in their sheep subjects with a discrimination procedure where only one of two stimuli was paired with shock. Neurotic subjects showed a higher and more irregular heart rate than normals in the experimental room, and gave an increase in heart rate to incidental stimuli whereas normals did not.

Moore and Marcuse (1945) ran two sows daily for 10 months using a tone CS and food UCS. They found a reliable increase in heart rate upon presentation of the CS, which preceded the UCS by 1 minute. Dykman and Gantt (1951) used a tone CS and a shock UCS, separated by 2 minutes, to produce an accelerative CR in dogs. As noted earlier, Zeaman and Wegner (1954), using a 2-second shock UCS, showed an increase in heart rate in human subjects with onset of the CS.

CS-UCS Interval and Regularity. Church and Black (1958) using dog subjects also found an accelerative CR with a tone CS and a 3-second shock UCS. Their results indicate that CR latency is shorter for a 5-second CS-UCS interval than for a 20-second CS-UCS interval. Latencies were virtually the same for the trace and delay conditioning procedures. No substantial differences in heart rate were observed between the various experimental treatments. This last finding is to be contrasted with some results of Bersh, Notterman, and Schoenfeld (1953) who found that an irregular time between CS and UCS produced more "anxiety" (i.e., heart rate CRs of greater magnitude) than a regular time between. A condition where shock did not always follow the CS produced more anxiety than either of these conditions.

Resistance to Extinction. One particular disclosure from the Soviet cardiac conditioning work seems to be of special importance (Bykov, 1957). That is, the CR developed in pairing a neutral stimulus with a pharmacological agent is very hard to extinguish. For example, some 296 presentations of the CS alone were required by Petrova to extinguish the cardiac CR.

Gantt (Bykov, 1957) reports that a cardiac conditioned reflex to food may persist 2 years after the salivary and motor components have been extinguished. Notterman, Schoenfeld, and Bersh (1952c) found that irregular pairing of the UCS with the CS gave greater resistance to extinction than regular reinforcement. They report further (1952a) that when subjects could avoid the shock UCS with a skeletal response, extinction was more rapid than when subjects were told there would be no shock in extinction. Both of these treatments produced more rapid extinction than the regular extinction procedure. In a later experiment (Bersh et al., 1956c) found that the CRs of subjects who were forcibly restrained from making the skeletal avoidance response extinguished more rapidly than the free avoidance subjects.

Generalization. Stimulus generalization of the CS has been demonstrated by Dykman and Gantt (1951) whose dog subjects differentiated between 256, 512, and 1,024 cps tones with respect to heart rate, latency, and EKG amplitude. Bersh, Notterman, and Schoenfeld (1956c) obtained generalization across tone frequencies as a function of intensity of the UCS. For a 28-volt alternating current shock UCS the human Ss showed a greater CR (depression of rate) and a flatter generalization across the 1,920, 1,020, 480, and 180 cps tones than for a 20-volt alternating current UCS.

CR across Trials. Heart rate conditioning data collected by Dawson (1953) are perhaps the best source of information for changes in the form of the heart rate CR across trials. They also illustrate sharply how deceptive a simple label such as a rate "increase" or "decrease" is in describing the cardiac CR. So far as such details are reported, most of the studies discussed earlier involved no more than 11 conditioning trials (e.g., Church & Black, 1958; Notterman et al., 1952b, 1952c; Zeaman & Wegner, 1954, 1958). In the Dawson experiment 20 conditioning trials were used and the second by second forms of the CR and UCR are shown for each five-trial block. These results show that the early CR is, in effect, an acceleration followed by a deceleration to the level preceding the CS. At this stage of conditioning a comparison of rates preceding and following the CS will show a net increase no matter which point within the CS-UCS interval is selected. As conditioning trials continue, however, the decelerative phase of the CR becomes more pronounced, such that rate of the heart cycles during this phase is less than the rate preceding the CS. Hence, increase or decrease in heart rate as *the* CR

depends heavily upon the location within the CS-UCS interval one uses, as well as the trial number (or number of trials if trials are averaged). We may then add these factors to others which affect the CR, such as UCS length, CS-UCS interval, and the kind and intensity of the UCS.

INTERACTION WITH OTHER BODY SYSTEMS

A factor which appears in elementary physiology texts suggests that the heart, as such, may not learn at all. This factor, obvious enough perhaps to be invisible, is respiration. Recent quantitative data clearly show how breathing may affect heart rate (Clynes, 1960; Huttenlocher & Westcott, 1957). Both inspiration and expiration produce a biphasic cardiac response: a brief accelerative phase followed by a decelerative phase of longer duration. This biphasic cardiac response is of greater magnitude and has a shorter latency for inspiration than for expiration (Clynes, 1960). Furthermore, it has been demonstrated that in a classical conditioning situation involving buzzer and shock, conditioned deep inspirations occur with the onset of the CS, and that the cardiac CR is a brief acceleration followed by a more pronounced deceleration (Huttenlocher & Westcott, 1957).

Regardless of which portion of the respiratory cycle might be correlated with the CS, there is the frightful prospect that cardiac conditioning work thus far has, in fact, been unknowingly concerned with respiratory conditioning. Or, with some luck, cardiac conditioning has merely been contaminated by the respiratory variable.

Fortunately, at least one cardiac conditioning experiment has been reported in which respiration was controlled. Westcott (1959) instructed subjects to breathe shallowly in time with a metronome during 10 CS (buzzer) alone trials and 10 conditioning trials when the CS and UCS (shock) were paired. The cardiac response in this experiment was a net drop in rate when the CS was given before conditioning, and a net increase in rate after the second conditioning trial. The conditioning curve was negatively accelerated across trials, showing an increase in heart rate over the pre-CS rate of 3.2 beats per minute on the last two trials. Respiration records showed consistent breathing on each trial, and across trials, for both frequency of respiration and the I/E ratios.

There are still other doubts about cardiac conditioning which we should consider. Kendon Smith (1954) argues that all conditioned visceral responses are in reality artifacts because they are brought on by activation of the skeletal musculature. According to this reasoning innate neural connections from the skeletal muscles activate the visceral systems with a muscular "bracing" to the UCS. Skeletal reactions are said to provide numerous afferent cues whereas "autonomic reactions generate no regulatory feedback whatever." Hence it is the skeletal system which is conditioned and the visceral system which merely accompanies. These ideas do badly in finding support from the cardiac literature discussing afferent pathways (e.g., Mitchell, 1956; Rushmer & Smith, 1959) for there is considerable anatomical evidence for autonomic feedback from the carotid and aortic bodies.

The opposite hypothesis, that skeletal responses can be mediated by autonomic responses is suggested by Wenzel (1959). Her data show an increase in heart rate to tones associated with food and a decrease to tones associated with shock. Whether or not heart rate differentiation between the two conditions is related to autonomic mediation of skeletal responses is yet to be shown in the laboratory.

Church and Black (1958) argue a similar case which is in line with Pavlov's "inhibition of delay." They too suggest autonomic mediation of skeletal responses. The tabulated latencies in their experimental report, however, tend to show shorter skeletal than autonomic latencies, which, after all, are consistent with the time constants of the two systems.

Perhaps the complexity of the organism is such as to preclude such simple cause and effect hypotheses about the various systems.

Conclusion

That the activity of the heart will change significantly in amplitude and rate in the presence of conditional stimuli is clear enough. There appear, however, to be mixed emotions as to the form of the heart rate CR since some authors report an increased rate, others a decreased rate, and still others either increased or decreased rate, depending on such factors as the UCR. The original question might then be what does the heart learn rather than does it learn? It is suggested that an answer to the second question may be found at two locations: at the desk, where heart rate changes would be treated as analog events rather than simple up or down events, and, at the laboratory, where like problems have previously been untangled with parametric study.

Some tentative principles have been abstracted from the papers reviewed:

1. Both form of the EKG cycle

and heart rate may be conditioned with the classical paradigm.

2. Latency of the heart rate CR is less for a shorter CS-UCS interval.

3. A CR of greater magnitude is produced when the UCS irregularly follows the CS.

4. CR resistance to extinction is great when some pharmacological UCSs are used. Resistance to extinction is increased with irregular CS-UCS pairings, and is decreased when UCS avoidance is made contingent upon a skeletal response.

5. There is a generalization gradient across tone frequencies as a function of UCS intensity.

6. The heart rate CR changes across trials such that the dominant accelerative portion of the response decreases as the decelerative portion increases.

Whether it is "really" the heart that learns, or something else such as the respiratory or the skeletal system, is perhaps a matter of degree. It seems unlikely that a particular bodily system is completely free from the influence of other bodily systems.

REFERENCES

ANDERSON, O. D., & PARMENTER, R. A long term study of the experimental neurosis in the sheep and dog. *Psychosom. med. Monogr.*, 1941, **2**(3–4).

BAINBRIDGE, F. A. The influence of venous filling upon the rate of the heart. *J. Physiol.*, 1915, **50**, 65–84.

BEIER, C. D. Conditioned cardiovascular responses and suggestions for treatment of cardiac responses. *J. exp. Psychol.*, 1940, **26**, 311–321.

BERSH, P. J., NOTTERMAN, J. M., & SCHOENFELD, W. N. The effect of randomly varying the interval between conditioned and unconditioned stimuli upon the production of experimental anxiety. *Proc. Nat. Acad. Sci., Wash.*, 1953, **39**, 553–570.

BERSH, P. J., NOTTERMAN, J. M., & SCHOENFELD, W. N. Extinction of human cardiac response during avoidance conditioning. *Amer. J. Psychol.*, 1956, **69**, 244–251. (a)

BERSH, P. J., NOTTERMAN, J. M., & SCHOENFELD, W. N. Generalization to varying frequencies as a function of intensity of unconditioned stimulus. *USAF Sch. Aviat. Med. Rep.*, 1956, No. 56–79. (b)

BERSH, P. J., NOTTERMAN, J. M., & SCHOENFELD, W. N. Relations between acquired autonomic and motor behavior during avoidance conditioning. *USAF Sch. Aviat. Med. Rep.*, 1956, No. 56–80. (c)

BERSH, P. J., NOTTERMAN, J. M., & SCHOENFELD, W. N. A comparison of internal vs. external reinforcement in motor avoidance situations. *USAF Sch. Aviat. Med. Rep.*, 1957, No. 57–27. (a)

BERSH, P. J., NOTTERMAN, J. M., & SCHOENFELD, W. N. The efficiency of pursuitrotor performance during experimentally induced anxiety. *USAF Sch. Aviat. Med. Rep.*, 1957, No. 57–28. (b)

BYKOV, K. M. *The cerebral cortex and the internal organs.* (Ed. & Trans. by W. H. Gantt) New York: Chemical Publishing, 1957.

CHURCH, R. M., & BLACK, A. H. Latency of the conditioned heart rate as a function of the CS-US interval. *J. comp. physiol. Psychol.*, 1958, **51**, 478–487.

CLYNES, M. Computer analysis of reflex control and organization: Respiratory sinus arrhythmia. *Science*, 1960, **131**, 300–302.

DAWSON, H. E. Concurrent condition of autonomic processes in humans. Unpublished doctoral dissertation, Indiana University, 1953.

DYKMAN, R. A., and GANTT, W. H. A comparative study of cardiac responses and motor conditioned responses in controlled "stress" situation. *Amer. Psychologist*, 1951, **6**, 263. (Abstract)

HUTTENLOCHER, J., & WESTCOTT, M. R. Some empirical relationships between respiratory activity and heart-rate. *Amer. Psychologist*, 1957, **12**, 414. (Abstract)

MITCHELL, G. A. G. *Cardiovascular intervation.* Edinburgh: Livingstone, 1956.

MOORE, A. U., & MARCUSE, F. L. Salivary, cardiac, and motor indices of conditioning in two sows. *J. comp. Psychol.*, 1945, **38**, 1–16.

NOTTERMAN, J. M., SCHOENFELD, W. N., & BERSH, P. J. A comparison of three extinction procedures following heart rate conditioning. *J. abnorm. soc. Psychol.*, 1952, **47**, 674–677. (a)

NOTTERMAN, J. M., SCHOENFELD, W. N., & BERSH, P. J. Conditioned heart rate response in human beings during experimental anxiety. *J. comp. physiol. Psychol.*, 1952, **45**, 1–8. (b)

NOTTERMAN, J. M., SCHOENFELD, W. N., & BERSH, P. J. Partial reinforcement and conditioned heart rate response in human subjects. *Science*, 1952, **115**, 77–79. (c)

OWENS, O., & GANTT, W. H. Does the presence of a person act on cardiac rate of the dog as unconditional stimulus? *Amer. J. Physiol.*, 1950, **163**, 746. (Abstract)

PATTERSON, S. W., PIPER, H., & STARLING, E. H. The regulation of the heart beat. *J. Physiol.*, 1914, **48**, 465.

RUSHMER, R. F. Applicability of Starling's law of the heart to intact, unanesthetized animals. *Physiol. Rev.* 1955, **35**, 138–142.

RUSHMER, R. F., & SMITH, O. A. Cardiac control. *Physiol. Rev.*, 1959, **39**, 41–68.

SKAGGS, E. B. Changes in pulse, breathing, and steadiness under conditions of startledness and excited expectancy. *J. comp. Psychol.*, 1926, **6**, 303–318.

SMITH, K. Conditioning as an artifact. *Psychol. Rev.*, 1954, **61**, 217–225.

WENZEL, B. M. Changes in heart rate associated with positive and negative reinforcement and their modification by reserpine. Paper read at the American Psychological Association, New York, September 1959.

WESTCOTT, M. R. The acquisition of a conditioned cardiac acceleration in humans. Paper read at Eastern Psychological Association, New York, 1959.

ZEAMAN, D., DEANE, G., & WEGNER, N. Amplitude and latency characteristics of the conditioned heart response. *J. Psychol.*, 1954, **38**, 235–250.

ZEAMAN, D., & WEGNER, N. The role of drive reduction in the classical conditioning of an autonomically mediated response. *J. exp. Psychol.*, 1954, **48**, 349–354.

ZEAMAN, D., & WEGNER, N. Strength of cardiac conditioned responses with varying stimulus durations. *Psychol. Rev.*, 1958, **65**, 238–241.

Voluntary Control of Human Cardiovascular Integration and Differentiation through Feedback and Reward

Gary E. Schwartz

The traditional notion of the autonomic nervous system is of a tightly controlled homeostatic network capable of little response separation or voluntary control. Contrary to this belief, recent research on instrumental learning of visceral responses has shown that individual functions can be brought under voluntary control and can show specificity of learning similar to that found for skeletal responses (*1*). For example, research on systolic blood pressure (BP) and heart rate (HR), two closely related autonomic responses, has shown that each can be separately controlled. (i) Providing human subjects with feedback and reward for increases or decreases in systolic BP leads to learned control of BP without corresponding changes in HR (*2, 3*). (ii) If increases or decreases in HR are reinforced, the subjects learn to control HR without similarly changing BP (*4*). Although this phenomenon has both theoretical and clinical importance (for example, as a potential treatment for decreasing specific symptoms in psychosomatic disorders), a suitable explanation for it has not yet appeared.

The purpose of the proposed integration-differentiation (ID) model (*5*) is to help provide a behavioral and bio-logical framework for understanding and predicting learned patterns of physiological activity. The model takes into account (i) the behavioral relations between responses as defined by the operant (feedback) procedure (*6*) and (ii) natural physiological changes or constraints that occur over time. In this context, the term integration is reserved for the response pattern in which two functions simultaneously change in the same direction (both increasing and decreasing together in a sympathetic-like pattern), and the term differentiation refers to the response pattern in which two functions simultaneously change in opposite directions (*7*). The first part of the model is an attempt to assess the activity of other physiological functions at the instant when a given physiological function is being reinforced, and the second part is an attempt to relate this information to naturally occurring changes in physiological activity due to stimulation, adaptation, and other factors not related to the contingency of reinforcement per se (*8*).

The general approach can be illustrated through a behavioral analysis of systolic BP and HR, two functions showing discrete bursts of activity that can be easily reduced to binary re-

SCIENCE, 1972, Vol. 175, pp. 90-93.

144

sponse units. With every heart contraction, BP rises and reaches a systolic peak, its magnitude determined by a complex interaction of HR, stroke volume, and peripheral resistance (9). If average (tonic) levels are specified for HR (in beats per minute) and for BP (in millimeters of mercury), each heart beat can be classified according to whether HR and BP values are above (^{up}) or below ($_{down}$) their tonic levels. At each heart beat only four coincidence patterns are possible: BP^{up} HR^{up}, BP_{down} HR_{down}, BP^{up} HR_{down}, and BP_{down} HR^{up}.

If the two functions naturally rose and fell together all of the time (BP^{up} HR^{up} and BP_{down} HR_{down} only), then even though an experimenter might select only one system for reward, he would unwittingly provide the same reinforcement for parallel changes in the other system. Accordingly, both functions would show simultaneous learning in the same direction (integration). At the other extreme, if the two functions always changed in opposite directions (BP^{up} HR_{down} and BP_{down} HR^{up} only), then when changes in one function were selected for reward, opposite changes in the other function would also receive contingent (100 percent correct) reinforcement. Again, both functions would show simultaneous learning, this time in opposite directions (differentiation). However, if the two functions were unrelated to the point of actually producing equal numbers of the four coincidence patterns, then when changes in one function were reinforced, the other function would receive a sequence of random reinforcement. (For example, if every BP^{up} was rewarded, HR would simultaneously be rewarded half the time for HR^{up} and half for HR_{down}.) Therefore, only the response receiving contingent reinforcement would be learned. I refer to this latter situation (when only the response chosen for reinforcement is learned) as specificity of learning.

My experiment was designed with two major purposes. One was to empirically determine the naturally occurring behavioral relationship between BP and HR, to test the hypothesis that, in order for specificity of BP and HR learning to occur, these two functions vary independently and thus go up and down together only about 50 percent of the time. The second aim was to answer the following question: if HR and BP (or any two functions) are randomly related, then is it possible to make them change together, or change in opposite directions? One implication of the ID model is that it should be possible to control a combination of functions, for example BP and HR, by rewarding the subject only when he shows the desired coincidence pattern of simultaneous changes in both functions (10). This procedure, although it reduces the percentage of correct reinforcement each function can receive (since neither function alone controls the reward), eliminates incorrect (undesired) rewards. A behavioral analysis would predict that if the frequency of the four coincidence patterns of BP and HR were equal and randomly distributed, then each pattern would show learning to the same degree. However, this prediction would fail if physiological constraints were preventing HR and BP from changing independently. In this case, the discrepancy between the predicted and measured extents of learning would uncover the ways in which the constraints were operating.

This approach requires a method for measuring on-line the phasic (beat-by-beat) and tonic (median) relationships between autonomic responses. Instrumentation was developed which determines at each heart beat the four coincidence patterns for BP and HR and also provides tonic value for each function during each trial (11) (Fig. 1).

Forty normotensive males (paid volunteers), 21 to 30 years old, were seated in a sound- and temperature-controlled room and connected to the physiological recording devices. Systolic BP, HR, and respiration were recorded on an Offner type R dynagraph. The electrocardiogram was measured with standard plate electrodes and displayed on one channel of the dynagraph. An electronic switch triggered Grason-Stadler (model 1200) solid-state programming equipment at each heart cycle (R spike of the electrocardiogram). The equipment automatically detected the four coincidence patterns for BP and HR and also presented all stimuli to subjects. Respiration was recorded by a strain gauge placed around the waist.

For each trial, median systolic BP was defined as the constant cuff pressure at which 50 percent of possible Korotkoff sounds occurred. Korotkoff sounds were displayed on one channel of the dynagraph in conjunction with a second electronic switch. With the use of this switch and of appropriate logic modules it was possible to count heart beats accompanied (within 300 msec) by a Korotkoff sound and heart beats not followed by a Korotkoff sound. Similarly, median HR was obtained by the use of a third electronic switch calibrated in beats per minute. The HR for each beat was displayed on one channel of the dynagraph through a cardiotachometer (Lexington Instruments model 107). With the use of appropriate logic modules in conjunction with the third (cardiotachometer) electronic switch, it was possible to count heart beats that were faster or slower than the value set by the cardio-

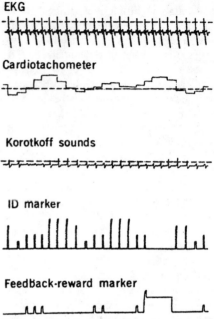

tachometer electronic switch.

Fig. 1. Representative portion of a polygraph record of the integration-differentiation (ID) system in operation. Shown are the electrocardiogram (EKG), heart rate (HR) displayed through a cardiotachometer, Korotkoff sounds measured at a constant cuff pressure, and two marker channels. Dashed lines represent the approximate levels of the three electronic switches. The presence or absence of a Korotkoff sound relative to the constant pressure in the cuff indicates whether blood pressure (BP) is up or down, while HR is rated up or down relative to the median HR. After each heart cycle (except during a reward) one of four possible marks appears on the ID marker channel. The longest and shortest marks indicate integration, with BP^{up} HR^{up} producing the longest mark and BP$_{down}$ HR$_{down}$ producing the shortest mark. The other two marks indicate differentiation, with BP^{up} HR$_{down}$ producing the third longest mark, and BP$_{down}$ HR^{up} producing the second shortest mark. The bottom channel indicates which one of the four possible combinations is eliciting feedback (short mark) and reward (long mark). In this example, feedback is occurring for BP$_{down}$ HR^{up} differentiation.

If Korotkoff sounds (BP^{up}) or fast heart beats (HR^{up}) or both exceeded the median levels by 35 in a given trial (50 heart beats in length), on the next trial the applied cuff pressure was raised 2 mm-Hg, or the cardiotachometer electronic switch was raised 2 beats per minute, or both changes were made. If the number of BP^{up} or HR^{up} or both exceeded the medians by less than 15 in a given trial, on the next trial the applied cuff pressure was lowered 2 mm-Hg, or the cardiotachometer electronic switch was lowered 2 beats per minute, or both changes were made. This shaping procedure made it possible to accurately track both BP and HR independently and simultaneously, and at the same time to obtain comparable information about relative changes in BP and HR at each beat.

Subjects were told that the purpose of the experiment was to determine whether they could learn to control certain physiological responses that are generally considered involuntary. They were instructed to refrain from moving and to breathe regularly. They were not told the nature of the specific responses to be controlled or the required directions of change. Twenty subjects were studied in two integration conditions. Half of these subjects received a 100-msec light and tone as feedback for each pulse cycle in which BP and HR simultaneously increased (BP^{up} HR^{up}); the other half received the same feedback each time their BP and HR simultaneously decreased (BP_{down} HR_{down}). Another 20 subjects were studied in two differentiation conditions. Half received the feedback only when their BP increased and their HR simultaneously decreased (BP^{up} HR_{down}), and the other half received the feedback for BP_{down} HR^{up} responses.

After giving every 12 correct responses, subjects were rewarded with a 3-second view of slides showing landscapes, attractive nude females, or cumulative bonuses earned (each slide was worth 5 cents). No feedback was given during the slides. All subjects receive 5 adaptation, 5 random reinforcement, and 35 conditioning trials. A blue light signaled the onset of random reinforcement and conditioning trials and remained on during the trials. Each trial was 50 heart beats long and was preceded by 10 seconds of cuff inflation. Intervals between trials ranged from 20 to 30 seconds; during this time the cuff was deflated. Subjects were matched according to their resting median BP's and randomly placed in one of the four conditions (12).

Figure 2 shows the average conditioning results for the four groups, based on the median cuff pressures and HR's obtained in each trial. Results are summarized as follows.

1) Subjects learned to directly integrate their BP and HR in a single session. Separate analyses of variance revealed highly significant group-by-trial interactions for BP ($P < .0001$) and HR ($P < .0001$), a result which indicates that the divergence of the two BP curves and of the two HR curves is reliable (13). Note that when BP^{up} HR^{up} is rewarded, both BP and HR increase somewhat and then return to baseline, while BP_{down} HR_{down} reinforcement yields sustained decreases in both. This result is very similar to earlier data obtained when each was separately rewarded (2, 4), except that in the present experiment control of both BP and HR is learned, and the learning effect is greater.

2) Integration was learned more easily than was differentiation. In fact, each of the integration groups earned more slides than either differentiation group. The divergence of the two BP curves in Fig. 2 (right) is reliable

($P < .0001$) and is very similar to the results for integration. In contrast, the divergence of the two HR curves in Fig. 2 (right) is not reliable, primarily because of the lack of sustained HR decreases in the BP^{up} HR_{down} group (13).

3) If the curves in Fig. 2 (left and right) are compared, the BP^{up} HR_{down} group is similar to the BP^{up} HR^{up} group, while the BP_{down} HR^{up} group is more similar to the BP_{down} HR_{down} group.

4) Clear evidence for learning of differentiation was obtained only for the BP_{down} HR^{up} group ($P < .0001$); the reverse pattern (BP^{up} HR_{down}) proved difficult to learn (14).

These results were anticipated from the ID model, by an analysis of the natural beat-by-beat and tonic relation of BP to HR during rest and during random stimulation in the present experiment and by a comparison of these data with earlier data on BP and HR

control (2–4). A summary of the predictions from the model follows.

1) The BP^{up} HR^{up} pattern would look as if it were learned less effectively than the reverse BP_{down} HR_{down} pattern, when the levels found at random stimulation were used as the standard. This prediction was based on data suggesting that systolic BP and HR tend to normally adapt (decrease relative to initial rest or random stimulation levels) during this type of experiment (2). Adaptation would therefore act to lower both the increase and decrease curves for BP and HR.

2) Tonic integration would be more readily learned than tonic differentiation. This prediction was based on the observation that median levels of BP and HR tend to increase (or decrease) together ($r = +.36$, $P < .05$) during the initial period of random stimulation. (For example, if a subject reacts to the beginning reinforcement trials

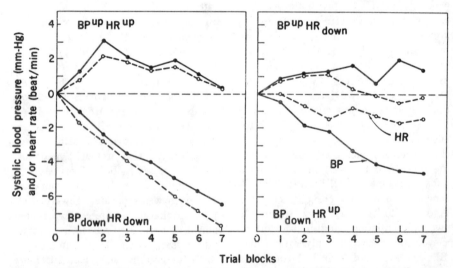

Fig. 2. Average systolic blood pressure (BP) and heart rate (HR) for the subjects being conditioned in the four coincidence patterns. On the left are data for the two integration conditions, on the right are data for the two differentiation conditions. Solid lines are BP, dashed lines are HR. Each point is the mean of five trials, set to zero by the last random trial. Beats per minute and millimeters of mercury are therefore on the same axis.

with a large tonic increase in BP, his HR will tend to show a comparable rise in level.) In other words, to the extent that the systems are tonically integrated in this experimental situation (other situations might heighten, eliminate, or possibly reverse this relationship), it should be easier to make them change together than in opposite directions.

3) Subjects reinforced for the BP^{up} HR_{down} pattern would raise both functions (and thus appear similar to the BP^{up} HR^{up} group); while subjects reinforced for the BP_{down} HR^{up} pattern would tend to lower both functions. This hypothesis is based on the following analysis of the BP and HR coincidence patterns. As predicted from the specificity findings (2–4), BP and HR change in the same direction only 53 percent of the time, and the frequency of the four coincidence patterns is approximately equal. However, close inspection of the coincidence patterns reveals that the relation between BP and HR over time is not truly random. Changes in HR precede those of BP; this relation produces a constant sequence of coincidence patterns (15). For example, the data indicate that when a BP^{up} HR^{up} pattern changes, 70 percent of the changes will be to a BP^{up} HR_{down} pattern. Therefore, to the extent that the BP^{up} HR^{up} pattern consistently precedes the BP^{up} HR_{down} pattern, then reinforcement for the latter will produce consistent (although delayed) reinforcement of the former as well. This is an example of a response chaining factor. Similarly, the data indicate that when a BP_{down} HR_{down} pattern changes, it will change with a 70 percent frequency to a BP_{down} HR^{up} pattern; this observation explains the similarity to BP_{down} HR_{down} learning when BP_{down} HR^{up} responses are reinforced. However, with natural tonic integration acting as a constraint, the

response chaining factor may have little influence when integration patterns for BP and HR (both increasing and decreasing) are directly reinforced.

4) The BP_{down} HR^{up} pattern would be more readily learned than the opposite BP^{up} HR_{down} pattern. This was predicted from the interaction of tonic and phasic factors in the present reinforcement procedure. To the extent that BP and HR normally adapt within a trial (but the electronic switches remain constant), the frequency of BP_{down} HR_{down} patterns would tend to increase toward the end of a trial. The BP_{down} HR^{up} pattern naturally occurs after a BP_{down} HR_{down} pattern, whereas the BP^{up} HR_{down} pattern rarely occurs after a BP_{down} HR_{down} pattern. In other words, it appears more feasible to change from a BP_{down} HR_{down} pattern by raising HR than by raising BP (16).

To test for conditioning of respiration during the experiment, analyses were made of respiration rate, variation of respiration rate, and variation of respiration amplitude. No differences were found between the four groups of subjects (17). Also, cognitive activity was assessed at the end of the experiment by a comprehensive questionnaire. Subjects in the BP_{down} HR_{down} group tended to check more items associated with relaxation than did the BP^{up} HR^{up} group, a result suggesting that some kind of arousal variable may have been operating. However, the two differentiation groups were indistinguishable from the BP^{up} HR^{up} group. Apparently, when a person is required to decrease the activity of more than one function simultaneously, subjective relaxation may occur.

Altogether, these data demonstrate that it is possible for human subjects to develop some control over the relation between their systolic BP and HR when they are provided with feedback and reward for the desired pattern of BP and HR. When the behavioral relation of these functions as "seen through the eyes of feedback and reward" is analyzed, and when natural biological constraints are taken into account, it appears possible to understand and predict the resulting pattern of learned control (18). To this extent, these results clarify earlier specificity findings and provide a new framework for research and theory in the control of multiautonomic functions. It is suggested that the present technique may be a tool for studying and controlling not only the relationship between visceral responses but the interaction of visceral responses with somatic and central behavior as well (19). This could be accomplished by assessing the extent and ease with which specific patterns of activity can be learned. The importance of considering feedback and reward in biological perspective is stressed, since natural physiological relationships and constraints do occur (20). It may be possible to apply these techniques to the treatment of specific clinical disorders; for example, to condition decreases in BP and HR to reduce the pain of angina pectoris (21).

References and Notes

1. For reviews of human research, see H. D. Kimmel, *Psychol. Bull.* 67, 337 (1967); E. S. Katkin and E. N. Murray, *ibid.* 70, 52 (1968). For reviews of animal research see N. E. Miller, *Science* 163, 434 (1969); L. V. DiCara, *Sci. Amer.* 222, 30 (January 1970).
2. D. Shapiro, B. Tursky, E. Gershon, M. Stern, *Science* 163, 588 (1969); D. Shapiro, B. Tursky, G. E. Schwartz, *Circ. Res.* 26-27 (Suppl. 1), I-27 (1970).
3. J. Brener and R. Kleinman, *Nature* 226, 1063 (1970).
4. D. Shapiro, B. Tursky, G. E. Schwartz, *Psychosom. Med.* 32, 417 (1970).
5. A complete description of the ID model and the present experiment can be found in G. E. Schwartz, thesis, Harvard University (1971).
6. For this report, no formal distinction is made between feedback (implying response information) and reinforcement (implying response contingency). Since both terms require experimental procedures for systematically producing changes in the environment which closely follow changes in behavior, their similarities (in obtained results) rather than differences (in theoretical underpinnings) are emphasized. Although I have primarily used the terminology developed in operant conditioning, feedback terminology can be easily substituted; the major implications and conclusions remain the same.
7. These definitions depart somewhat from those generally used in biology, where the term integration refers to any consistent pattern of unified activity, regardless of direction, while differentiation refers to a separation of one response from others (here called specificity).
8. For example, if a response decreases naturally from the beginning to the end of an experiment this changing operant baseline must be taken into account to measure the direction and extent of learning. See A. Crider, G. E. Schwartz, S. R. Shnidman, *Psychol. Bull.* 71, 455 (1969).
9. R. F. Rushmer, *Cardiovascular Dynamics* (Saunders, Philadelphia, 1961).
10. A similar approach has been used to train rats to differentially control blood volume between the two ears. See L. V. DiCara and N. E. Miller, *Science* 159, 1485 (1968).
11. A preliminary experiment on learned cardiovascular integration in which the procedure was tested can be found in G. E. Schwartz, D. Shapiro, B. Tursky, *Psychosom. Med.* 33, 57 (1971).
12. No subjects showing initial systolic blood pressures of 135 mm-Hg or more during the last adaptation or random reinforcement trial were included in this experiment.
13. Analyses of variance were performed on an IBM 360 computer with the Biomed 08V program. Groups was the between factor and trials was the within factor. The degrees of freedom for the group by trial interaction was 34/612. For the BP data, the analyses of variance (comparison of two groups at a time; six possible combinations) revealed that over trials the two BP^{up} conditions were each significantly higher than each of the two BP_{down} conditions ($P < .0001$), but were not different from each other. For HR, all two-group comparison trials were significant ($P < .01$ to .0001) except $BP^{up} HR^{up}$ with $BP^{up} HR_{down}$, and $BP^{up} HR_{down}$ with $BP_{down} HR^{up}$. The corresponding group main effects for these comparisons were also significant for BP ($P < .025$ to .005) and HR ($P < .10$ to .0001).
14. For example, separate analyses of variance on each of four groups, with measures (2) (change in BP versus change in HR) and trials (35) as within factors, indicated that $BP_{down} HR^{up}$ reinforcement was the only condition that produced a reliable divergence between BP and HR during trials (d.f. = 34/306).
15. Sinus arrhythmia, a condition in which HR leads BP, is discussed by A. M. Scher, in *Physiology and Biophysics*, T. C. Ruch and H. D. Patton, Eds. (Saunders, Philadelphia, 1965), p. 660.
16. This pattern of results is also consistent with physiological theory suggesting that the parasympathetic system is capable of finer dif-

ferentiation than is the sympathetic system. Raising the HR while lowering the BP may constitute a parasympathetic pattern, since HR may be increased by a decrease in vagal tone. Unlike elevation of HR, elevation of systolic BP requires sympathetic activity, hence the observed difficulty in lowering HR at the same time.

17. Finer analysis procedures (for example, co-incidence measures of BP, HR, and respiration) may be necessary to assess such effects.
18. Predictive power of the ID model will, by definition, be limited to the extent that (i) operant (feedback) theory adequately handles the learning of individual responses (the interaction of other variables such as cognitive set and motivation is yet little understood); and (ii) physiological mechanisms and constraints can be empirically assessed in the given situation.
19. The recently published report by E. E. Fetz and D. V. Finocchio [*Science* 174, 431 (1971)], which demonstrates operant conditioning of specific patterns of neural and muscular activity in the monkey, strongly supports this view.
20. For example, when changes at each beat in diastolic (as opposed to systolic) BP are reinforced, some conditioning of HR also takes place (D. Shapiro, G. E. Schwartz, B. Tursky, *Psychophysiology*, in press). This implies that diastolic BP and HR are partially (but not completely) integrated with respect to phase. Analysis of BP^{up} HR^{up} and BP_{down} HR_{down} coincidence responses has confirmed this prediction (average phasic integration is 70 percent). Research is required to determine the extent to which these two integrated functions can be separated through operant differentiation reinforcement (for example, requiring the subject to decrease diastolic BP by reducing peripheral resistance, while at the same time increasing HR).
21. The circumstances under which cardiac oxygen requirements in angina pectoris can be reduced if both HR and BP are lowered are discussed by E. Braunewald, S. E. Epstein, G. Glick, A. A. Wechsler, N. H. Wechsler, *N. Engl. J. Med.* 277, 1278 (1967); E. H. Sonnenblick, J. Ross, E. Braunewald, *Amer. J. Cardiol.* 22, 328 (1968).
22. Supported by NIMH research grant MH-08853; research scientist award K5-MH-20,476; ONR contract N00014-67-A-0298-0024; and the Milton Fund of Harvard. I especially thank D. Shapiro and B. Tursky for guidance and encouragement, and J. D. Higgins for comments on the manuscript.

Hypnotic Control of Peripheral Skin Temperature: A Case Report

Christina Maslach,

Gary Marshall, and Philip G. Zimbardo

ABSTRACT

In an exploratory study on the specificity of autonomic control, subjects attempted to simultaneously change the skin temperature of their two hands in opposite directions. Subjects who were trained in hypnosis were successful in achieving this bilateral difference, while waking control subjects were not. These findings demonstrate the powerful influence that cognitive processes can exert on the autonomic nervous system and also suggest the possibility of more effective therapeutic control of psychosomatic problems.

DESCRIPTORS: Hypnosis, Skin temperature, Autonomic control, Psychosomatic medicine.

Maintenance of a relatively constant level of body temperature is a vital physiological function. It is so efficient and automatic that we become aware of the process only when pathological internal conditions cause us to react with fever or chills, and when extremes of environmental conditions markedly alter the skin temperature of our limbs. To what extent can such a basic regulatory function be brought under volitional control?

Luria (1969) performed an experiment dealing with this question, in which he studied the mental feats of a man with eidetic imagery. Apparently, his subject could induce such vivid visual images that they exerted a profound influence on his behavior. When he was instructed to modify the skin temperature in his hands, he was able to make one hand hotter than it had been by two degrees, while the other became colder by one and a half degrees. These bilateral changes were attributed by the subject to the "reality" of his visual images, which consisted of putting one hand on a hot stove while holding a piece of ice in the other hand. Is such a phenomenon replicable with "normal" individuals not born with the remarkably developed eidetic ability of this man? We were led to believe so on the basis of converging research findings in the areas of visceral learning, cognitive control of motivation, and hypnosis.

Neal Miller and his associates at Rockefeller University (1969a, 1969b) have

This study was financially supported by an Office of Naval Research grant NOOO 14-67-A-0112-0041 to Philip G. Zimbardo, supplemented by funds from an NIMH grant 03859-09 to Ernest R. Hilgard.

PSYCHOPHYSIOLOGY, 1972, Vol. 9, pp. 600-605.

recently demonstrated that the control over skeletal muscle responses through operant conditioning procedures can be extended to responses of the glands and viscera. Their work has generated the powerful conclusion that any discriminable response which is emitted by any part of the body can be learned if its occurrence is followed by reinforcement. These results are extended in the work of Zimbardo and his colleagues (1969) which experimentally demonstrates that biological drives, as well as social motives, may be brought under the control of cognitive variables such as choice and justification, even in the absence of external reinforcers.

It appeared to us that hypnosis: a) is a state in which the effects of cognitive processes on bodily functioning are amplified; b) enables the subject to perceive the locus of causality for mind and body control as more internally centered and volitional; c) is often accompanied by a heightened sense of visual imagery; and d) can lead to intensive concentration and elimination of distractions. For these reasons, it should be possible for well-trained hypnotic subjects to gain control over regulation of their own skin temperature without either external reinforcement or even external feedback. While there have been some attempts to control temperature through hypnosis or other methods (Barber, 1970; Green, Green, & Walters, 1970), they have often lacked adequate controls and tend to focus only on unilateral changes.

Our present study was exploratory in nature and attempted to demonstrate that hypnotic subjects would be able to achieve simultaneous alteration of skin temperature in opposite directions in their two hands, while waking control subjects would not. The bilateral difference of one hand becoming hotter than normal, while the other gets colder, was chosen in order to rule out any simple notion of general activation or prior learning and to control for any naturally occurring changes in skin temperature. We also attempted to rule out other alternative explanations of changes in skin temperature by keeping environmental conditions constant and by minimizing overt skeletal responses on the part of the subjects.

Method

Subjects

All of the subjects (with the exception of the junior author—PGZ) were undergraduate paid volunteers from the introductory psychology course at Stanford University. Three of the Ss received hypnotic training prior to the experiment, while the remaining 6 Ss did not. The training averaged about 10 hrs per person and was usually conducted in small groups. It was permissive in orientation, stressing the S's ability to achieve self-hypnosis, and involved several criterion tests.

Procedure

The Ss were individually tested in the Laboratory of Dermatology Research at the Stanford Medical Center. The ambient temperature in this room was automatically regulated to maintain a constant level. Ten thermocouples of copper constantin were taped to identical sites on the ventral surface of the two hands and forearms of the S. Both room and skin temperatures were continuously monitored by a Honeywell recording system. The Ss lay on a bed with their arms resting comfortably at their sides and with open palms extended upward in exactly the same position. This posture was maintained throughout the session. and there was no overt body movement.

For the hypnotic Ss, the experiment began with approximately 10 min of hypnotic induction. The remainder of the session was identical for both hypnotic and waking control Ss. They were first asked to focus attention on their hands, and were then told to make an arbitrarily selected hand hotter, and the other colder, than normal. Accompanying this last, brief instruction were suggestions of several images which could be useful in producing this effect, as well as encouragement to generate personal imagery and commands which might be necessary to achieve the desired result. The S lay in silence for the duration of the testing session (which averaged about 10 min). The final instruction was to normalize the temperature in both hands by returning it to the initial baseline level. Each of the Ss participated in 2 such sessions. In addition, 1 of the Ss completed 2 sessions utilizing auto-hypnosis, a procedure in which the S provides the instructions to himself.

Results

All of the hypnotic Ss demonstrated the ability to produce bilateral changes in skin temperature. Large differences (as much as 4° C) between identical skin sites on opposite hands appeared within 2 min of the verbal suggestion, were maintained for the entire testing period, and then were rapidly eliminated upon the suggestion to normalize skin temperature. Temperature decreases in the "cold" hand were generally much larger than the increases in the "hot" hand, the largest decrease being 7° C, while the largest increase was 2° C. In contrast, none of the waking control Ss were able to achieve such significant bilateral changes in the temperature of their hands. Any temperature change that they did exhibit was usually in the same direction for both hands (rather than in opposite directions), thus yielding close to a zero score for bilateral change (see Fig. 1). The difference between these control scores and the consistently large bilateral changes of the hypnotic Ss is highly significant ($t = 14.27$, $df = 7$, $p < .001$). All of the hand thermocouples reflected these successful bilateral changes, while

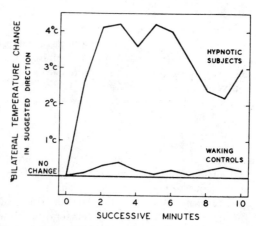

Fig. 1. Mean algebraic sum of bilateral skin temperature differences ("successful" directional changes in each hand were weighted positively, while changes which were opposite to the suggested direction were weighted negatively).

154

the forearm thermocouples showed no temperature changes at all, thus indicating the specificity of this hypnotic control process. Also, the performance of the hypnotic Ss showed an improvement from the first to the second session; this was not true of the control Ss.

When the individual patterns of reaction in the hypnotized Ss are examined, the degree of control that they were able to exert becomes even more apparent. The S's data shown in Fig. 2 reveals how, following the suggestion to make her left hand colder and right hand hotter (opposite to their relative baseline position), she rapidly "drove" them in the appropriate directions. After maintaining the separation for more than 10 min, she re-established the initial baseline difference as soon as she was given the instruction to normalize her skin temperature. Since there was no overlap in the temperature distributions of the two hands, the obtained differences from min 4 to min 16 were extremely significant (within-subject $t = 20.18$, $df = 12$, $p < .001$).

Both the hypnotic and waking control Ss reported trying hard to meet the experimental demand. Several of the control Ss even believed that they had successfully completed the task, although as noted earlier, their largest bilateral difference was very slight. All Ss also reported that they had generated assorted imagery to help them produce changes in their skin temperature. Some of the

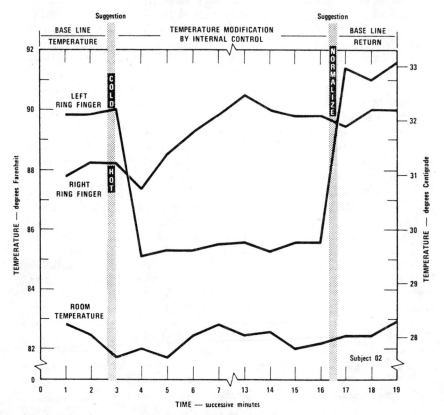

Fig. 2. Simultaneous modification of skin temperature in opposite directions in the right and left hands (omitted min 8–12 are no different from the rest of the modification period).

imagery involved realistic experiences, such as having one hand in a bucket of ice water and the other under a heat lamp, while other imagery had a more symbolic or fantasy quality. In addition, *Ss* also used image-less "commands" given independently to each hand (i.e. "you become hot, you become cold").

In the initial pre-test, verbal feedback was given to the *Ss* when they had succeeded in producing the bilateral difference in temperature. Such feedback had an unexpected negative effect, resulting in the "loss" of the attained difference, and was subsequently eliminated in the experimental sessions. It may be that the intensive concentration required to achieve the unusual performance demanded in this study was disturbed by having to attend to and process the informational input from the experimenter. In a sense, the feedback, although supportive, operated as a distractor to attenuate the obtained differences in skin temperature. The ability of hypnotic *Ss* to successfully perform this task without feedback is particularly evident in the data of the *S* using auto-hypnosis, who was able to produce bilateral differences in skin temperature without the aid of any external demands, feedback, or extrinsic sources of reinforcement.

Discussion

Although we are not in a position to characterize the underlying physiological mechanisms responsible for the bilateral control of skin temperature which we have shown, we believe that the role of hypnosis in the process is quite understandable. The research by Miller on visceral learning has stressed the important function served by curare in paralyzing the skeletal musculature of the animals. At first, this methodological control was thought to be necessary only to rule out possible influences of skeletal musculature on glandular and visceral responding. However, it now appears that curarizing the animals "may help to maintain a constant stimulus situation and/or to shift the animal's attention from distracting skeletal activities to the relevant visceral ones [Miller, 1969b, p. 19]."

We would argue that the effects of hypnosis are analogous to those of curare, since hypnosis provides a set of training conditions which permit a greater than normal degree of generalized relaxation, removal of distracting stimuli, and enhanced concentration upon a given, relevant dimension. Hypnotic training may also aid in the control of experiential, behavioral, and physiological processes by increasing the subject's confidence in his ability to exert such control, and by altering consciousness to the point that words and images can be more readily translated into a code language to which he is physiologically responsive.

To us, the significance of research in this area is less in understanding how hypnosis per se operates, but rather how human beings "naturally" learn to induce ulcers, tachycardia, excessive and uncontrolled sweating, and other forms of psychosomatic illness. Miller's work suggests that the intervention and modification of such reactions follow principles of operant conditioning. Our work adds the possibility that the sources of reinforcement in both producing and changing psychosomatic symptomatology may be cognitive in nature. In a recent clinical application of these ideas,[1] patients are trying to reduce their migraine headaches by learning how to voluntarily control their blood flow and skin temperature via biofeedback techniques. Therapeutic control may thus be best achieved by com-

[1] Sargent, J. D., Green, E. E., & Walters. E. D. Unpublished research report entitled. "Preliminary Report on the Use of Autogenic Feedback Techniques in the Treatment of Migraine and Tension Headaches," 1971.

bining the precision of reinforcement contingencies with the power of a more pervasive cognitive approach to dealing with such mind-body interactions.

REFERENCES

Barber, T. X. *LSD, marihuana, yoga and hypnosis*. Chicago: Aldine Publishing Co., 1970.

Green, E. E., Green, A. M., & Walters, E. D. Self-regulation of internal states. In J. Rose (Ed.), *Progress of cybernetics: Proceedings of the International Congress of Cybernetics, London, 1969*. London: Gordon and Breach, 1970.

Luria, A. R. *The mind of a mnemonist*. New York: Discus Books, 1969.

Miller, N. E. Learning of visceral and glandular responses. *Science*, 1969, *163*, 434–445. (a)

Miller, N. E. Autonomic learning: Clinical and physiological implications. Invited lecture at the XIX International Congress of Psychology, London, 1969. (b)

Zimbardo, P. G. *The cognitive control of motivation*. Glenview, Ill.: Scott, Foresman and Co., 1969.

157

PART V

PLASTICITY OF PSYCHO-MOTOR COMPETENCY

CAUSES OF RETARDATION AMONG INSTITUTIONAL CHILDREN: IRAN

WAYNE DENNIS[1]

A. INTRODUCTION

Considerable interest has recently been shown in the fact that in some institutions for children there occurs a decided retardation in behavioral development. The observations of Spitz (8, 9, 10) in particular have received much notice, chiefly because of the interpretations which Spitz has placed upon his data. In our opinion, the primary importance of these observations lies in their challenge to the theory that infant development consists largely of the maturation of a motor sequence which is little affected by learning.

Aside from the investigations of Spitz, studies of behavioral retardation among institutional children have been few in number. The scarcity of such studies is due in large part to the fact that institutions in which conditions comparable to those described by Spitz can be found are not numerous. In many countries institutional care has been replaced by other methods of caring for dependent children. However, institutions in which behavioral development is retarded can still be found in countries which are "underdeveloped" not only in regard to modern technology but also in respect to newer methods for the care of foundlings and other homeless infants.

The present paper reports studies of development in three institutions in Tehran, the capital of Iran. In two of these institutions, children are exceedingly retarded in their motor development. In the third little retardation is present. It is believed that comparisons of child care in these institutions,

[1] This study was conducted during 1958-1959 when the author was on leave from Brooklyn College and served as a visiting professor at the American University of Beirut, Lebanon. The investigation was made possible by a grant from the Rockefeller Brothers Fund to the American University of Beirut, and by a grant to the author from the Social Science Research Council. In Tehran, the assistance of Miss Gay Currie of the U.S.P.H.S. and I.C.A. was invaluable. The institutions in Tehran participating in the study were most coöperative; they have not been named in this report but can readily be identified by persons acquainted with the local scene. Special thanks are due to Mrs. B. Azuri who served as interpreter and research assistant. The manuscript has greatly benefited from the suggestions and criticisms of colleagues at the American University of Beirut and at Brooklyn College.

JOURNAL OF GENETIC PSYCHOLOGY, 1960, Vol. 96, pp. 47-59.

and of behavioral development in them, will throw considerable light upon the nature of the environmental factors which influence motor development. This paper supplements a recent report on behavioral retardation in a Lebanese institution by Dennis and Najarian (4). In the earlier report attention was directed primarily to motor development in the first year of life, whereas in the present instance the period from one year to four years of age is the one with which we are mainly concerned. Preliminary observations indicated that development during the first year in the two Iranian institutions in which retardation occurs is essentially the same as in the Lebanese institution described in the previous paper. For this reason in the present study attention is given chiefly to the age period to which little attention was directed in the earlier report.

B. Description of the Institutions

The two institutions in which marked retardation occurs, which will be called Institutions I and II, are supported chiefly by public funds; the third institution, to be labeled III, is supported by private funds. Several other children's institutions both public and private, exist in Tehran. The present report should not be taken to imply that retardation prevails in the majority of Iranian institutions.

It is worthy of note that the number of children to be found in institutions in Tehran is quite large. This number is explained by several factors. For one thing, Tehran is a large city, having approximately two million inhabitants. The recent growth of Tehran has taken place in the main through migration from villages. This has led to a considerable amount of social disorganization which has increased the number of illegitimate children, foundlings, abandoned children, orphans and half-orphans. Furthermore in Tehran at the present time, provisions for the care of dependent children, other than by institutionalization, are quite inadequate. Consequently, almost all children not living with parents or relatives are to be found in institutions.

1. *Institution I*

Institution I feels obligated to accept all foundlings and all abandoned children under three years of age who are brought to it. The population of the institution varies from day to day because of departures and admissions. During the time of the present study (September, 1958) the average daily population was about 600; of these about 275 were between birth and one year of age, 135 were between one and two years of age, and about 110 were between two and three years of age. While children above three years are generally transferred to other institutions, a few remain in Institution I beyond this age.

The excess of younger children over older children in Institution I may be due to several causes, including an increased intake rate in recent years, a higher death rate during the first year than in later years, return of older children to relatives, and transfer of older children to other institutions. The data at our disposal do not permit an assignment of relative weights to these factors.

More than nine-tenths of the children in Institution I are recorded as having been under one month of age at the time of their admission. When the actual date of birth is not known, an estimate of age at admission, based on weight, size, and appearance is made and placed in the child's record.

The mother never accompanies the child to Institution I nor sees him after admission.

In general children are placed in individual cribs, although at times, because of over-crowding, two infants temporarily occupy the same crib. In such instances, the heads of the two babies are placed at opposite ends of the bed.

A child is bathed on alternate days. Except when being bathed, the younger children spend practically their entire time in their cribs. They are given milk and other liquids while lying in bed, the bottle being supported by a small pillow. When semi-solid foods are introduced, infants are sometimes held by an attendant and sometimes fed in bed. The children are placed in bed in the supine position. They are never placed prone and seldom get themselves into this position.

The paucity of handling is due primarily to the attendant-child ratio. On the average there were eight children per attendant. In addition to feeding the children, bathing them, and changing clothing and diapers, the attendants are also responsible for changing the bed-linen and cleaning the rooms, and have some responsibilities for preparing food. Each attendant is on duty 12 hours per day. In general there are 32 children and four attendants to a room, although this varies somewhat according to the size of the room. There is no assignment of attendants to particular children. The attendants have no special training for their work and are poorly paid. The emphasis on the part of the supervisors seems to be on neatness in the appearance of the rooms, with little attention to behavioral development.

In his crib the child is not propped up, and is given no toys. The child who can pull himself to sitting, and hence is in some danger of falling from his shallow crib, is placed, when awake, on a piece of linoleum on the composition stone floor of the room. Until he himself achieves the sitting position he remains in bed. In two rooms some of the children who can sit are seated in a row on a bench which has a bar across the front to prevent falling. Aside from these two benches and the frames for the cribs, the rooms have no children's furniture and no play equipment of any kind.

2. *Institution II*

This institution accepts children over three years of age. The children in this institution come mainly from Institution I. Child care practices in II are a continuation of the practices existing in I, but sanitation and cleanliness are poorer and the appearance of the children suggests that nutrition and health are poorer. However, in neither I nor II are there any records of growth in height or weight, and it was not possible for us to obtain any objective assessment of nutritional status.

3. *Institution III*

Institution III was established only one year prior to the present study. It was started primarily to demonstrate improved methods of institutional care. The children in III come from Institution I but are selected for transfer in the early months of life. It seems likely that those sent to Institution III are chosen from among the more retarded children. They remain in III until three years of age unless adopted before that date. The number of children per attendant is 3–4. Children are held in arms while being fed, are regularly placed prone during part of the time they are in their cribs, are propped up in a sitting position in their cribs at times and are placed in play pens on the floor daily when above four months of age. Numerous toys are provided. Attendants are coached in methods of child care, and supervisors emphasize behavioral development as well as nutrition and health.

Individual growth charts are available for each child in Institution III and show without exception that these children are much below prevailing weight norms on arrival but attain normal weight within a few months.

C. Types of Behavioral Data

Quantitative observations on the behavioral status of the groups described above were made only with regard to motor coördinations. Some general observations on social and emotional behavior will be presented after motor behavior has been discussed.

In respect to motor development, each child who was a subject of this study was classified with regard to his ability to meet each of the following behavioral criteria:

1. *Sit alone.* The child was placed in a sitting position on the floor. He was scored as sitting alone if he maintained this position for one minute. However, if a child could maintain this position at all he ordinarily could maintain it indefinitely.

2. *Creep or Scoot.* The child was placed sitting on the floor and was encouraged to locomote by having the attendant hold a cookie, or extend her arms, toward the child at a distance of about six feet. He was scored as passing the test if he covered the distance in any manner. If he locomoted, his mode of progression was recorded. The modes of locomotion will be discussed at a later point.

3. *Stand by holding.* The child was held under the arms and placed adjacent to the horizontal bars of a child's bed. It was observed whether or not he grasped the bars and maintained a standing position.

4. *Walk by holding.* The child who could stand by holding was observed for some minutes to determine whether he took steps while holding. He was urged to walk by the attendant.

5. *Walk alone.* The child who could walk by holding objects was placed standing without support and was encouraged to walk to the outstretched arms of the attendant. The child was scored as walking alone if he took at least two steps without support.

In the above tests one of the attendants with whom the child was familiar was coached to make the tests while the experimenter remained at a distance of six feet or more from the child and somewhat behind him. This procedure was followed because it was found that the child's unfamiliarity with the experimenter often inhibited the child's behavior if he was tested by the examiner himself. Communication between the attendant and the examiner was conducted via an Iranian interpreter. Tests were conducted among the children of a given room only after the experimenter and the interpreter had made several visits to the room and somewhat decreased the children's shyness. If a child failed a test, the attendant was asked whether or not he could usually perform the required response. If the answer was positive, renewed efforts were made to elicit a successful performance. The experimenter is convinced that subjects who were scored as failing a test were actually unable to perform the required task.

The numbers of children tested at each age level in each institution are shown in Table 1. In Institutions I and II the total number of children tested was 123. In selecting children to provide this sample, the children of appropriate ages were selected at random from each of several rooms, the rooms so far as we could determine not being unusual in any respect. However, we excluded from testing any child who had sensory or motor defects, who was ill or who had recently been ill. In Institution III all children between age one and three were tested. They totaled 51.

TABLE 1
PER CENT OF EACH GROUP PASSING EACH TEST

Institutions	I	I	II	III	III
N	50	40	33	20	31
Ages	1.0-1.9	2.0-2.9	3.0-3.9	1.0-1.9	2.0-2.9
Sit alone	42	95	97	90	100
Creep or Scoot	14	75	97	75	100
Stand holding	4	45	90	70	100
Walk holding	2	40	63	60	100
Walk alone	0	8	15	15	94

D. RESULTS OF TESTS

Table 1 shows the per cent of each group which passed each test. The reader is asked to direct his attention first to the retardation which is evident in Institutions I and II. Among those children in Institution I who were between 1.0–1.9 years of age, fewer than half could sit alone and none could walk alone. In normative studies, of home-reared children, such as those conducted by Jones (6), Gesell (5), Dennis and Dennis (2) and others, it has been found that by nine months of age all normal non-institutional American children can sit alone. By two years of age nearly all can walk alone. A majority of the children of Institution I cannot perform these responses at ages at which almost all home-reared children can perform them. It will be noted that even between 2.0–2.9 years of age only 8 per cent of the children in Institution I are able to walk alone and only 15 per cent of those children in Institution II who are 3.0–3.9 years of age are able to walk alone. We are not aware that any groups so retarded as Groups I and II have previously been reported.

In Institution III the picture is different. Of those children between 2.0–2.9 years of age nearly every child is able to walk unaided. While these children do not equal the performance of home-reared children, their motor behavior is much superior to that of children in Institutions I and II. In other words it is not institutionalization per se which handicaps Groups I and II since Group III children who are also institutionalized are but slightly retarded in motor development. The records of Group III also show that motor retardation is not a general characteristic of Tehran children.

Of special note is the difference in types of pre-walking locomotion between Institutions I and II on the one hand and Institution III on the other.

165

Of the 67 children in Institutions I and II who engaged in creeping or scooting, only 10 did so by creeping, i.e., going on hands and knees or on hands and feet. All others progressed by "scooting," i.e., their locomotion took place in the sitting position, the body being propelled forward by pushing with the arms aided by propulsion from the legs. Many children who could not walk were quite adept at scooting.

Since tests for creeping or scooting were made when the child was in a sitting position, it might seem that the frequency of scooting was due to the nature of the starting position. To test the effect of starting position, many subjects who were "scooters" were placed prone and offered a cookie at some distance, a powerful incentive for locomotion in these children. In each case the child first pushed himself to a sitting position and then scooted. Scooting was definitely the preferred mode of locomotion even when the child was placed prone. So far as we could determine, the majority of the scooters were completely unfamiliar with creeping.

In Institution III, the reverse situation prevailed. Of 15 children who were observed to creep or scoot, all progressed by creeping. No scooting whatsoever was seen in this institution, yet tests were made from the sitting position as with Groups I and II. When placed sitting and encouraged to locomote, the children leaned forward, got themselves on hands and knees, and crept.

E. INTERPRETATIVE COMMENTS ON MOTOR DEVELOPMENT

Let us examine now the probable reasons why the children in Institutions I and II were so severely retarded relative to home-reared children and why they were so much more retarded than children in Institution III. Several different possibilities need to be considered.

Attention should first be directed to malnutrition as a possible cause of retarded motor development. As noted earlier there can be no doubt that many of the children in Group I were much smaller and lighter than non-institutional children and children of the same age in Group III. There can be no doubt, too that malnutrition can be so severe as to interfere with motor performance and motor progress. But the question at stake is not whether malnutrition can affect motor functions but whether malnutrition was in fact a major cause of the retardation of Groups I and II.

We are inclined to think that undernourishment was not the major factor. The following considerations have led us to this interpretation: In the first place, Groups I and II were not entirely listless and inactive. In this connection we need to bring out a fact that we have not noted in earlier sec-

166

tions, namely that these children engaged to a considerable extent in auto-matisms such as head shaking and rocking back and forth. In many cases, these actions were quite vigorous. These activities tend to indicate that these children were not slow in motor development simply because of motor weakness.

The second consideration is somewhat similar to the first, namely, that the locomotor activities in which the children in Groups I and II engaged seem to require as much as or more energy than the locomotor activities which are usual at their respective ages, but in which they did not engage. For example, while few two-year-olds in Group I walked, three-fourths of them locomoted, chiefly by scooting. No physiological data are available, but it seems likely that the metabolic cost of covering a certain distance by scooting is as great as, or even greater than, the effort required to go the same distance by walking. Certainly this would be true for an adult, but of course one cannot argue from the adult to the child. At any rate the possibility exists that the reason that these children scooted was because this was the only form of locomotor skill which they had learned, not that they were too weak to walk.

This interpretation seems to be borne out by the fact that the pre-walking methods of locomotion were different in different groups. The retarded groups scooted. It is difficult to believe that malnutrition can lead to scooting rather than creeping. It is far from obvious that scooting is "easier" than creeping. If it is, why should not all children choose the easier method? In other words, the differences between groups seem to us to be due to the outcome of different learning situations rather than to differences in nutri-tional status.

What were the differences in the situations faced by Groups I and II and Group III which may account for the development of two different types of locomotion and different degrees of retardation? We suggest the following:

In Group III and in many homes infants are propped up in a sitting position, or held in a sitting position. In this position the child can raise his head and can partially raise his shoulders for short periods and can relax these efforts without falling. He can thus practice some elements of sitting. On the other hand, the child who remains on his back has no such opportuni-ties to learn to sit. In some respects it is surprising that children who are never propped up or held on the lap are able to learn to sit at all. But it will be remembered that in Groups I and II some children could not sit until they were more than two years of age. Until they could sit alone, all forms of locomotion were impossible for them, because they were not placed in a position in which creeping was possible.

This is not true in Group III. In this group and in many homes, the child is frequently placed prone in bed or on the floor. In this position he can raise his head from the surface, push with his arms, raise his chest, pull his arms and legs beneath his body—in other words, he can practice acts which are employed in creeping. The child who lies on his back nearly every moment of the day is denied such practice. Thus one specific item of child care, i.e., occasionally placing the child face downward, may well contribute to the development of creeping in most children and its absence may account for the lack of creeping in Groups I and II.

The question may be raised as to why children in Institutions I and II did not get themselves into the prone position in their cribs. Repeated observations of these infants in their cribs showed that few ever attained the prone position. The probable reasons are the small size of the cribs and the softness of the beds, both of which made turning over very difficult.

It is likely that this item, i.e., absence of placement in the prone position, may lead to delayed development not only in regard to creeping but also in respect to walking. The child who can creep can go to a piece of furniture, grasp it and pull to his knees. This may lead to walking on his knees while holding furniture. Many children go from knee walking to walking by holding to furniture and thence to walking alone. In contrast to the child who creeps, the child who scoots to a piece of furniture is sitting when he arrives at his goal and can attain a higher position only by lifting his entire weight by his arms. In our opinion, the lack of creeping accounts in large measure for the retardation in walking of Groups I and II.

We are well-aware that some persons have interpreted the behavioral retardation of institutional infants to emotional factors rather than to a paucity of learning opportunities. Some have even suggested that under certain conditions institutional infants simply "waste away" from psychological, not from medical causes, a process called marasmus.

If marasmus actually exists, it has somehow been escaped by several hundred children in Iranian institutions living under conditions which are supposed to foster it. Although the prevailing emotional tone of children in Institutions I and II is dysphoric, it is difficult to conceive of mechanisms whereby their unhappiness retards their motor development and causes them to scoot rather than to creep.

There remains the necessity of relating the results of the present study to certain findings reported earlier by the present author. We refer to a study which found no apparent effect of cradling upon the motor development of Hopi children (3) and a study which indicated that infant development can proceed normally under conditions described as "minimal social stimulation" (1). On the surface these results seem contradictory to those here reported, because the former studies found that environmental deprivations had but little effect whereas the present study reports that major consequences can ensue from them. In fact, however, the studies are not contradictory but complementary. To bring the results of these studies into harmony, one needs only to examine the kinds of deprivation which were involved and their severity. Certain differences among these studies seem to us to be crucial. The Hopi children were limited in regard to learning opportunities only *while on the cradleboard*. As we pointed out in our original report, they were on the cradleboard chiefly during these sleeping hours, when in any case little learning is expected to occur. When awake they were handled, held upright against the mother, placed sitting on her lap, and placed prone. Their deprivation of learning opportunities was much less than that encountered by the children in Institution I who 24 hours per day for many months remained in a supine position.

A similar contrast exists between Rey and Del, the subjects of an experiment in environmental deprivation, and children in Institutions I and II. Rey and Del were not deprived to the same degree nor in the same manner as the institutional children described above. As the original report shows (1), Del and Rey, beginning at nine months, were regularly placed in a prone position on a pad on the floor. After it was found that they could not sit alone they were given special practice in sitting. Del and Rey were also given special training in supporting their weight when held upright. Such training was not given in Institutions I and II.

These experiences with special training given to Del and Rey suggest that the retardation of the institutional children could be fairly rapidly remedied if intensive specialized practice were given them. Unfortunately it was not possible for us to undertake such experiments while we were in Tehran. The speed with which delayed skills can be developed remains an important problem for future researches with institutional children.

So far as the permanency of motor deficiencies is concerned it should be noted that Institution II had many children between ages 6 and 15 years who presumably were as retarded at ages two and three as were the children whose behavior was described above. Yet these children were attending school, playing games, doing chores, and being trained in difficult skills, such as the weaving of Persian rugs. There was nothing in their general behavior to suggest that any permanent consequences issued from the extreme retardation in motor development during the early years. To be sure, we have no direct evidence that these children were retarded at two and three years of age, but so far as we could ascertain there has been no change in the child care offered by Institutions I and II and no reason to suppose that their early development was different from that of their counterparts in the present study.

Finally let us note that the results of the present study challenge the widely-held view that motor development consists in the emergence of a behavioral sequence based primarily upon maturation. Shirley's chart of the motor sequence is a textbook favorite. It shows sitting alone at seven months, creeping at 10 months, and walking alone at 15 months. The present study shows that these norms are met only under favorable environmental conditions. Among the children of Institution I not only was sitting alone greatly retarded but in many cases creeping did not occur. Instead, an alternate form of locomotion was employed. These facts seem to indicate clearly that experience affects not only the ages at which motor items appear but also their very form. No doubt the maturation of certain structures, which as yet cannot be identified, is necessary before certain responses can be learned, but learning also is necessary. Maturation alone is insufficient to bring about most post-natal developments in behavior. This is also the conclusion which we reached in the Del-Rey experiment, but the present study supports this position more dramatically because the limitations of learning in Institutions I and II are more drastic and more long-continued than were those in the Del-Rey study.

F. Social and Emotional Behavior

Only incidental observations were made relative to social and emotional behavior. Several of these had to do with the infants' reactions to visitors.

In the weeks preceding our tests, it appears that Institution I seldom had visitors. The children of Institution II formerly had few visitors but several weeks before our arrival a volunteer social service group, aware of the isolation of these children, began to make periodic visits to them, taking them from their beds, holding them, and carrying them about. Institution III also had several visitors, partly because of the demonstration nature of this orphanage.

Children in Institution I, probably because of their unfamiliarity with visitors, were somewhat afraid of us during our first visit. They did not smile with us and, in most cases, would cry if we picked them up. On repeated visits, however, they became more friendly, smiled at us, and before our work was completed some of them would hold out their arms to be carried.

Most of the children in Institution II were positive to visitors at the beginning of our work. Several employed attention-seeking devices before visitors and cried if other children were selected for attention. In contrast in Group III, probably because of the greater time spent with attendants and because of their familiarity with visitors, there was little fear of strangers and only limited attention seeking.

Eagerness for food appeared to be greatest in Institution II. In this institution there was much crying before meal time. Children of this group handled cups and spoons quite well. In general there was very little wasting of food on the part of these children. Cups of milk were reached for eagerly, handled carefully, and drunk rapidly. There were attempts, sometimes successful, on the part of those who had finished eating to obtain the food of others, and hitting, pinching, and biting were sometimes the outcomes of such clashes. Children who could not walk could nevertheless manage to attack others and to defend themselves with considerable skill. After feeding they became much more jovial and nearly every child could be made to smile or laugh by an adult who shook him lightly or tickled him.

G. Summary

This paper has presented data concerning behavioral development among 174 children, aged one year to four years, in three Iranian institutions. In Institutions I and II infant development was greatly retarded. The behavioral progress of children in the third institution was much less retarded. The interpretations offered for these differences in behavior among the children of different institutions are as follows: the extreme retardation in Institutions I and II was probably due to the paucity of handling, including the failure of attendants to place the children in the sitting position and the prone position. The absence of experience in these positions is believed to have retarded the children in regard to sitting alone and also in regard to the onset of locomotion. The lack of experience in the prone positions seems in most cases to have prevented children from learning to creep; instead of creeping, the majority of the children in Institutions I and II, prior to walking, locomoted by scooting. In Institution III, in which children were frequently handled, propped in the sitting position, and placed prone, motor development resembled that of most home-reared children. The retardation of subjects in Institutions I and II is believed to be due to the restriction of specific kinds of learning opportunities. This interpretation was found to be congruent with the results of other studies in environmental deprivation. In the light of these findings, the explanation of retardation as being due primarily to emotional factors is believed to be untenable. The data here reported also show that behavioral development cannot be fully accounted for in terms of the maturation hypothesis. The important contributions of experience to the development of infant behavior must be acknowledged.

REFERENCES

1. DENNIS, W. Infant development under conditions of restricted practice and of minimum social stimulation. *Genet. Psychol. Monog.*, 1941, **23**, 143-189.
2. DENNIS, W., & DENNIS, M. G. Behavioral development in the first year as shown by forty biographies. *Psychol. Rec.*, 1937, **1**, 349-361.
3. ————. The effect of cradling practices upon the onset of walking in Hopi children. *J. Genet. Psychol.*, 1940, **56**, 77-86.
4. DENNIS, W., & NAJARIAN, P. Infant development under environmental handicap. *Psychol. Monog.*, 1957, **71**, 1-13.
5. GESELL, A. Infancy and Human Growth. New York: Macmillan, 1928.
6. JONES, M. C. The development of early behavior patterns in young children. *Ped. Sem.*, 1926, **33**, 537-585.
7. SHIRLEY, M. M. The First Two Years: Vol. I. Postural and Locomotor Development. *Inst. Child Welfare Monog. Series*, No. 6. Minneapolis: Univ. Minn. Press, 1933.
8. SPITZ, R. A. Hospitalism, an inquiry into the genesis of psychiatric conditions in early childhood. *Psychoanal. Stud. Child*, 1945, **1**, 53-74.
9. SPITZ, R. A. Hospitalism: A follow-up report. *Psychoanal. Stud. Child*, 1946, **2**, 113-117.
10. SPITZ, R. A. Anaclitic depression. *Psychoanal. Stud. Child*, 1946, **2**, 313-342.

PERCEPTUAL-MOTOR ABILITIES OF DISADVANTAGED AND ADVANTAGED KINDERGARTEN CHILDREN

ENNO S. LIETZ

Summary.—On individually administered perceptual-motor tests, 50 advantaged kindergarten children performed significantly better than 50 disadvantaged kindergarten children. Also, boys performed as well as girls and the white and black disadvantaged children performed equally well except on perceptual-motor match.

Many articles have been written about the characteristic environment of a deprived child. Such factors include the lack of books, magazines, toys, and even father absence from the home is considered a variable. How important a role each one of these variables has upon the child has never been determined. However, they all seem to be closely related to family income. It is for this reason that family income has been used as a criterion in the legal definition of an economically disadvantaged child by the State of Illinois. If a child is part of a family which has an income of 3000 dollars a year or less, he is eligible for the special programs funded by the state. Since this study was conducted in the state of Illinois, and Ss were part of this funded program, the term "disadvantaged child" refers to a child who comes from a home where the family income is 3000 dollars or less per year.

It was the purpose of this study to examine the perceptual-motor abilities of the kindergarten child and determine if a significant difference exists between the disadvantaged children and those from families whose income is above the designated poverty level. The term "advantaged" applied to the children who came from homes where the income was above the poverty level.

If one is to assume that effects of early sensory deprivation have caused the disadvantaged child to begin with an inferior set of cognitive skills as compared to his middle-class counterpart, then ways to narrow this gap must be sought. The general question is whether the perceptual-motor skills of the disadvantaged children are significantly different from those of the advantaged. Also, if there is any difference in these skills, in what areas from a developmental point of view might one anticipate that girls would score higher than boys in perceptual-motor tests. Therefore, sex differences were assessed in addition to racial ones.

During the past decade many studies of environmental deprivation of young children have been made. Spitz (1946) and Goldfarb (1945) have indicated the very serious consequences of early sensory deprivation in later life. Comparison by Skeels (1965) of institutionalized children and those placed in foster homes showed that environmental stimuli have a great impact on the intellectual development of a child. Fowler's work (1962) indicated that early intervention with the stimulus-deprived child will produce changes conducive to greater success in school achievement. In addition to institu-

PERCEPTUAL MOTOR SKILLS, 1972, Vol. 35, pp. 887-890.

tionalized children, slum area children also lack the environmental stimuli as pointed out by Bruner (1966). Studies by John and Goldstein (1964) indicate that concept formation, visual discrimination, language acquisition, and IQ are related to the amount of social and physical deprivation or enrichment concomitant to the child's status on each of three dimensions.

Research on perceptual training is recent and isolated findings have not always been well received. But much of the work is favorable to introducing such training. Witkin (1960) and Bolger (1952) lend support to perceptual training and their work indicates that intellectual growth, improved coordination, and motor activity may result from perceptual training.

METHOD

Of 100 Ss whose age ranged from 64 to 75 mo., 50 were from economically disadvantaged homes where the annual income was less than $3,000 and 50 were from a middle-class home environment. There were approximately the same number of boys and girls in each group. The 50 disadvantaged children were in a preschool program in the racial strife-torn city of Cairo, Illinois. Many parents were attending school to be retrained for a new occupation. Father's absence was common. The 50 advantaged children were from a kindergarten in a nearby community of Staunton, Illinois. Fathers of these children worked in factories or were school teachers or local merchants.

A revision of the *Purdue Perceptual-motor Survey* by Roarch and Kephart (1966) was individually administered. Included in this revised form were nine of the original 30 subtests which were selected with the help of the author of the original test, Dr. Newell C. Kephart. Dr. Kephart stated he has used these nine subtests with kindergarten students and established their validity and reliability. Four major areas in perceptual-motor development were measured with these nine subtests, balance and posture, body image and differentiation, perceptual-motor match, and form perception. The four areas were described by Kephart (1960).

Subtests 1, 2, and 3 used a walking beam which was the wide side of a 2-in $\times$ 4-in., 10-ft. board, placed 6 in. off the floor. Test 1 required walking the board forward, Test 2, walking it sideways and Test 3, walking it backwards. These tests measured balance and posture.

Two subtests measured body image and differentiation, with jumping on one foot and then both feet, followed by skipping and then hopping. The other subtest consisted of playing the old game of "Angels in the Snow." This test is a modification of a childhood game where the child lies in the snow and moves his arms and legs. The child lies on his back and is asked to make various movements with his arms and legs. This test seems to be particularly useful in detecting problems with right or left-sidedness

The area of perceptual-motor match was tested by using chalkboard activities. The child was asked to draw a circle at the blackboard with chalk and also to draw a line between two points placed on the board in front of him by the testor.

Form perception required copying four forms, the circle, cross, square, and triangle. Organization of the copied forms on the paper was inspected. Administering the test to 100 children required about 20 school days. As kindergarteners had a short day, about 5 to 7 students a day were tested. The administration and evaluation of each performance was accomplished by using Roarch and Kephart's (1966) directions and criteria. The examining areas were away from the classrooms to minimize copying or imitative behavior by other children. It was assumed that intelligence, like perceptual-motor ability, was randomly distributed in the samples.

RESULTS AND DISCUSSION

An analysis of variance, three-dimensional design, was used to examine differences between the boys and girls in the disadvantaged and advantaged groups. The first test was of triple interaction ABC as shown in Table 1 to determine if the corresponding interaction effects of two of the factors differ in magnitude from level to level of the third factor. Upon finding no triple interaction, the statistical design permitted testing for double interactions and main effects.

TABLE 1
SUMMARY OF ANALYSIS OF VARIANCE OF SCORES ON PERCEPTUAL-MOTOR SKILLS BY ADVANTAGED AND DISADVANTAGED GROUPS

Sources	df	MS	F	p
A (Advantaged-Disadvantaged)	1	251.250	151.62	.05
B (Boys-Girls)	1	6.100	3.68	
C (Perceptual-motor Areas)	3	1616.540	975.58	.05
AB	1	3.470	2.09	
AC	3	14.740	8.89	.05
BC	3	.093	.05	
ABC	3	1.644	.99	
Within Cells	384	1.657		
Total	399			

A nonsignificant BC interaction between sex and perceptual-motor area indicated that the relative effects for boys and girls were the same in each of the four areas. A nonsignificant AB interaction (Table 1) indicated that the boys and girls performed relatively the same whether advantaged or disadvantaged. Boys appear to be able to perform perceptual-motor skills as well as girls. No further comparisons were made. Since there was no first-order interaction found for the sample tested, the main effects of sex could be tested. A nonsignificant F (Table 1) indicated there was no difference in the perceptual-motor skills of boys and girls.

The second hypothesis concerned the possible difference in the perceptual-motor ability of the black and white disadvantaged children. Table 2 shows the t ratio for these measures was 1.85, which did not reach the level (1.96) required for $p_{.05}$. Apparently racial differences were not important unless one were willing to accept $p_{.10}$. Under the circumstances it seemed wise to look at the various areas for differences (see Table 3). Since the degrees of freedom for

TABLE 2
PERCEPTUAL-MOTOR ABILITY OF NEGRO AND WHITE DISADVANTAGED CHILDREN

Group	N	M	S^2
Negro	28	23.14	15.69
White	22	25.18	12.51

TABLE 3

Analysis of Variance of Means for Negro and White Disadvantaged Children in Perceptual-Motor Skills

Sources	df	SS	MS	F	p
Balance and Posture					
Treatments	1	1.02	1.02	.27	
Groups Within	48	179.46	3.73		
Total	49	180.48			
Body Image and Differentiation					
Treatments	1	.10	.10	.20	
Groups Within	48	23.98	.49		
Total	49	24.08			
Perceptual-motor Match					
Treatments	1	17.58	17.98	10.65	.05
Groups Within	48	79.60	1.65		
Total	49	97.18			
Form Perception					
Treatments	1	9.05	9.05	3.46	
Groups Within	48	125.43	2.61		
Total	49	134.48			

these four tests were the same (Table 3), the tabled value of F, 4.08 at $p_{.05}$, was the same for all four tests. Only one test, perceptual-motor match, showed a significant difference, with the black children scoring significantly lower. Why this occurred cannot be answered by the present data but should be pursued.

REFERENCES

BOLGER, H. H. An experimental study of the effects of perceptual training on group IQ scores of elementary pupils in rural ungraded schools. *Journal of Educational Research*, 1952, 63, 43-53.

BRUNER, J. The cognitive consequences of early sensory deprivation. In G. R. Hawkes & J. L. Frost (Eds.), *The disadvantaged child.* Boston: Houghton Mifflin, 1966. Pp. 137-144.

FOWLER, W. Cognitive learning in infancy and early childhood. *Psychological Bulletin*, 1962, 59, 116-152.

GOLDFARB, W. Effects of psychological deprivation in infancy and subsequent stimulation. *Psychological Review*, 1945, 102, 18-23.

HEBB, D. O. The effects of early experience on problem solving at maturity. *American Psychologist*, 1947, 11, 306-307.

JOHN, V. P., & GOLDSTEIN, L. S. The social context of language acquisition. *Merrill-Palmer Quarterly*, 1964, 10, 265-276.

KEPHART, N. C. *The slow learner in the classroom.* Columbus, O.: Merrill, 1960.

ROARCH, E. G., & KEPHART, N. C. *The Purdue Perceptual-motor Survey.* Columbus O.: Merrill, 1966.

SKEELS, H. M. Effects of adoption on children from institutions. *Children*, 1965, 12, 33-34.

SPITZ, R. A. Analclitic depression: an inquiry into the genesis of psychiatric conditions in early childhood. *Psychoanalytic Study of the Child*, 1946, 2, 313-342.

THOMPSON, W. R., & HERON, W. The effects of restricting early experience on the problem-solving capacities of dogs. *Canadian Journal of Psychology*, 1954, 8, 17-31.

WITKIN, H. A. The problem of individuality in development. In B. Kaplin & S. Warner (Eds.), *Perspectives of psychological theory.* New York: International Univer. Press, 1960. Pp. 60-74.

PART VI

A PROPOSAL FOR A COMPREHENSIVE VIEW OF PSYCHO-MOTOR DEVELOPMENT

PSYCHO–MOTOR COMPETENCE
AND THE
ANISA PROCESS–CURRICULUM

Linda M. Blane and Daniel C. Jordan
Center for the Study of Human Potential
University of Massachusetts

The general mobility of man and his power to execute
an extremely wide variety of bodily movements make him
unique among all living creatures. Development of a bipedal means of locomotion left his fore limbs free to
manipulate objects. Equipped with a special kind of hand
--four fingers with an opposable thumb--man was not only
able to become an expert tool-user, but also able to
become the kind of thinker who can invent no end of new
tools (Whitehead, 1967). But thoughts are intimately
related to speech and speech requires the coordination of
a large number of fine movements of muscles which make up
the diaphragm, mouth, tongue, face, larynx, and pharynx.
Thus man's ability to control and coordinate these muscles
was indispensable to the transmission of cumulative knowledge from one generation to the next through language.
Such knowledge, in turn, increased his powers of survival
through the establishment of ever-enlarging cooperative
social units. But the story does not end there. Man's
extraordinary psycho-motor endowment had other far-reach-
ing implications for his continuing development because it
enabled him to interact with his environment in more complex ways than any other animal [1], thus providing him with
the diversity of stimuli that compelled him perpetually to
modify himself as well as the environment external to him.

---

[1]The Anisa theory of development defines development
as the translation of potentiality into actuality. A
basic proposition of the theory establishes interaction
with the environment as the primary means by which the
translation is sustained. See Appendix for overview of
the Anisa theory of development and curriculum.

ORIGINAL MANUSCRIPT, 1974.

The number of different accomplishments which has resulted
from such movement capability is evident today not only in
the range of types of work in which man is engaged, but is
also apparent in a wide variety of recreational activities
and performing arts. A champion skater, a skilled balle-
rina, a virtuoso violinist, vocalist or pianist, a trapeze
artist, basketball player, acrobat, juggler, cardsharp,
neuro-surgeon, high diver, and judo expert--none of these
fails to impress us with the variety, complexity, and high
degree of refinement of the movements of which the body and
its parts are capable.

But precisely what has movement of muscles to do with
education, outside of learning particular muscular skills?
Whitehead sensed its general significance:

> I lay it down as an educational axiom that
> in teaching you will come to grief as soon
> as you forget that your pupils have bodies
> ... . The connections between intellect-
> ual activity and the body, though diffused
> in every bodily feeling, are focussed in
> the eyes, the ears, the voice and the hands
> (Whitehead, 1967).

A large number of studies have yielded an extensive
body of information about psycho-motor development which
confirms Whitehead's educational axiom. Approaches to
these studies reflect different frames of reference. The
medical researchers (Gesell, 1948), physical education
specialists (Cratty, 1970), and to some extent psychologists (Bayley, 1945; McGraw, 1943; and Shirley, 1931), have
been responsible for the wealth of normative data, some
developed from longitudinal studies. With the exception of
Cratty and his students, physical educators have been primarily concerned with accuracy and efficiency of movements
as adjusted to particular activities--gross and fine motor
skills and their expression in sports and games.

Many of the research efforts which have resulted in
normative, age-related data provide important information
about developmental sequences, but are not sufficient to
explain them and their interrelations. Because they do
not directly facilitate the identification and explication
of processes which constitute the development of psycho-
motor competence, these data are limited in their usefulness.
Furthermore, they do not explain conditions which enhance
or inhibit the growth of psycho-motor competence. Thus,

they offer little that is directly usable by the teacher or teacher educator concerning experience which can best promote psycho-motor competence at each stage in an individual child's development.

Other research efforts have begun to provide information on developmental processes, indicating that development follows orderly and relatively fixed sequences. These studies also confirm that the rate of development for an individual may vary according to internal (maturational) and external factors (variety of stimuli and an environment which provides opportunities for movement). Some of them have contributed to a growing body of evidence that there is a strong relationship between the emergence of psycho-motor competence and perceptual (Conway, 1974), cognitive, affective, and volitional competence. We have drawn on them liberally in formulating the Anisa theory of development and have used them to document the identification of processes which underlie learning competence in the psycho-motor area. It is important to note that in the Anisa model learning is very broadly defined and includes far more than simply the storage of verbally-coded information. Coordination and control of the movement and position of muscles is a fundamental and indispensable form of learning. Thus, the processes whereby psycho-motor potentialities are actualized form an important category in the process-curriculum of the model. Understanding the nature of these processes depends upon knowledge of the skeletal structure, the nature of different kinds of muscles and how they are activated by nerves.

BONES, MUSCLES, AND NERVES

Bones

At the time of puberty the skeleton of the body is comprised of some 350 separate bony masses which are reduced to a final total of 206 in the adult through the process of fusion. These bones are held together by ligaments and form a complex system of levers operated by muscle fibers which are activated by electro-chemical impulses transmitted by a complex network of nerves. The types of movements possible by any complex of interrelated bones is determined by the nature of the joints among them. There are three basic kinds of joints: (1) hinge joints which have only one axis of rotation (i.e., knee); (2) joints with two axes of rotation (i.e., occipital bone of

the skull as it is articulated with the atlas); and,
(3) joints with three axes of rotation--ball and socket
joints (i.e., articulation between scapula and humerus or
shoulder joint).

Muscles

From the middle layer of differentiating cells in the
embryo, the mesoderm, skeletal and muscular structures
emerge. By the end of eight weeks, these structures and
their interconnections have reached a stage of development
where elementary functioning is possible. Studies carried
out on embryos and fetuses delivered by Caesarian section
have established that the human embryo can respond to
tactile stimuli by contracting its muscles. By the time
of the fourth intrauterine month, a number of specific
reflexes can be identified. As the neural-muscular basis
for the movement of particular muscles develops, the intrauterine child will exercise many of them. Thus, a great
deal of motor learning takes place before birth. In
particular, sucking and breathing movements are practiced
in utero.

The child is born with a finite number of muscle
fibers and for all practical purposes acquires no new ones.
Thus, increase in the size of particular muscles is due to
an increase in the size of the individual fibers compris-
ing the muscle rather than an increase in the number of
fibers. During the pre-school period, growth of muscle
tissue constitutes between one fourth and one third of the
total body weight. During the early years, muscle is composed of around 72% water and 28% solids. These percentages change significantly during puberty, when the
proportion of solid material increases and the percentage
of water decreases. Because of the high water content in
children's muscles, muscle fatigue sets in quickly and the
child tires easily. For these reasons, a great deal of
sleep and sufficient rest is required for normal development.

There are three basic kinds of muscle: (1) skeletal
muscle, (2) smooth muscle, and (3) cardiac or heart muscle.
Skeletal muscles are attached to bones by tendons and
ligaments and are responsible for moving different body
parts through a complicated system of levers. Skeletal
muscle fibers have different contractile characteristics,
some contracting more slowly thereby fatiguing less easily

while others contract much more quickly and therefore fatigue more rapidly. Any given muscle may contain both types of fibers or be predominately of one type. Muscles which maintain posture, for instance, have a large number of muscle fibers which contract more slowly and therefore fatigue less easily. Smooth muscle is found within the walls of viscera, around glands, and in the walls of blood vessels. Contraction spreads from one fiber to the next in ways that are much slower in comparison to contraction rates of skeletal muscle. Cardiac muscle comprises the greatest part of the heart.

Each of these different kinds of muscle has cellular structures that are quite different and the means of innervation are also different. The skeletal muscles are most capable of voluntary control, smooth muscles to a lesser extent, and cardiac muscle least of all. Psycho-motor competence means gaining maximum voluntary control to whatever degree is possible over all muscles regardless of the category to which they belong. However, the manner in which control is gained differs with each category.

Nerves

How the billions of embryonic nerve fibers manage to reach their appropriate destinations in muscles, tendons, joints, glands, and sensory receptors is one of the great unsolved developmental mysteries. Somehow, all of the right connections are made and all muscles properly supplied with appropriate nerve endings thereby readying the total bodily structure for active functioning. The complexity of the network of the nervous system with particular reference to the termination of nerves in muscle fiber taxes the imagination. In brief, motor nerves leave the spinal cord and eventually reach skeletal muscles. Each nerve entering a muscle divides into a large number of smaller branches each of which terminates on the surface of a single muscle fiber. Thus, a single motor nerve supplies a number of skeletal fibers. The one nerve cell and the muscle fibers supplied by it form a motor unit. An impulse traveling through the nerve will excite the contraction of all the muscle fibers connected to it. Any one muscle may be comprised of a large number of motor units. In man, some individual muscles have fewer than one hundred muscle fibers per motor unit while others may have up to two thousand. Muscles with a large number of motor units for a given number of muscle fibers are subject to a more refined control than a muscle which has only a few motor units for the same number of muscle fibers. For instance, the thumb is moved by muscles which have many small units each one of which has only a very few muscle fibers; thus, the thumb is capable of highly refined and controllable movements. By comparison, the anti-gravity muscles (muscles which resist the pull of gravity on the body, mostly in the legs and back) have fewer motor units each of which has a large number of muscle fibers.

The innervation of smooth muscles is not fully understood. Every smooth muscle fiber does not necessarily have a nerve terminating in it and it is uncertain how such fibers are controlled. However, it is known that, although a great deal of smooth muscles apparently cannot be brought under voluntary control, with careful exercise and practice, some of them can. It is possible, for instance, to learn how to reduce blood pressure by voluntarily relaxing the muscles in the walls of blood vessels. Dealing with high blood pressure in this way has many advantages over the use of drugs to achieve the same ends.

The cardiac muscle has a specialized supply of nerves from the autonomic nervous system. They are stimulated by fibers of the sympathetic division of the autonomic nervous system and are inhibited by fibers from the parasympathetic division of the autonomic nervous system. There is very little direct voluntary control possible over the cardiac muscle although it is possible to learn how to reduce or speed up heart rate voluntarily.

Up to this point we have spoken only of nerves which carry impulses from the central nervous system to the muscles. There are also nerves which carry impulses from muscles to the brain. Embedded in muscles, tendons, and joints are special sensors called proprioceptive receptors. Different kinds of receptors convey different kinds of information to the brain. Among the most important receptors are neuro-muscular spindles which are sensitive to changes in tension and provide information to the brain about how much a muscle is being stretched (instantaneous length) and the velocity of the stretch. Other kinds of receptors which appear in tendons are stimulated by tension produced in the tendon when muscles either contract or stretch. Receptors are also present in connective tissue around muscles and bones, particularly in the joints. All of the receptors in non-skeletal muscles seldom provide feedback that reaches a level of conscious awareness although this can be increased with particular kinds of practice.

To summarize, the muscular system is activated through nerve impulses, much of which can come under voluntary control through learning. The types of movements which can be executed are limited by the kinds of bones and joints to which they are attached (Gardner, 1958). Psycho-motor competence is determined by the extent to which movement and coordination of muscles come under volitional control. Coming under such control is the translation from potentiality of movement to the actuality of competent muscular actions. An individual who has difficulty making this translation will not only achieve less psycho-motor competence, but may have difficulty in developing competence in other areas. Because development in all areas is sustained by interaction with the environment, ability to move oneself and manipulate the environment also has implications for the emergence of perceptual, cognitive, volitional, and affective competence.

DEVELOPMENTAL TRENDS

In general, development refers to a progressive increase in complexity of the organization of structures and their related functions. In the case of psycho-motor development, organization proceeds through the following general phases:

1. Undifferentiated mass activity/reflex activity.

2. Differentiation of movements.

3. Integration of movements into patterns.

4. Generalization of different movement patterns to a variety of similar situations or tasks.

In addition to the above, development also proceeds in accordance with three other over-arching patterns which give direction to the processes of differentiation, integration and generalization. These over-arching patterns are discernible in development as it proceeds in cephalo-caudal (head to tail) and proximo-distal (from the center of the body outward to the ends of the limbs) directions. Gross motor movements are differentiated, integrated, and generalized prior to fine motor movements; thus, there is an

overall developmental pattern from gross to fine. Finally,
there is a trend from bilaterality to unilaterality, usually
resulting in dominance of one side over the other. This
one-sidedness results in right-handedness or left-handedness.
The same is also true for the legs and feet (e.g., we tend
to kick a ball consistently with either the right or the
left foot).

Undifferentiated Mass Activity/Reflex Activity

Even though he is extremely active, the newly born child
is able to coordinate very few motor responses voluntarily.
This early period is one of undifferentiated mass activity.
Yet this activity is not unrelated to what is going on in
the environment. Abrupt or intense stimuli will produce an
increase in the mass activity whereas caressing or other
kinds of gentle stimuli will tend to reduce it. In the midst
of the undifferentiated mass activity, several coordinated
and specific responses are discernible--the newborn child's
unlearned reflexes. These reflexes are regulated by numerous spinal and subcortical nerve centers which are suffi-
ciently developed to be functional at the time of birth.
The child has little or no control over these movements;
they occur automatically in response to specific stimuli.
Such reflexes include movements of the muscles of the face,
mouth, diaphragm, throat, digestive system, eyelids, eyeballs,
and certain foot, leg and arm responses. From this undifferentiated mass activity and the reflexive patterns present
a birth, the development of voluntary differentiated and
coordinated muscular activity emerges.

Differentiation of Movements

Out of the confusion of waving limbs and sensory input,
the infant begins to distinguish differences in muscles and
the forces necessary to activate them. This separation of
one muscle from another eventually results in increasing control over the movement of body parts. Probably one of the
first efforts at control occurs when the infant moves his
head in a specific direction to enable his eyes to see a
desired object or to locate an object from which a sound is
coming. The child, in performing such a coordinated movement, has mastered a complex series of muscular acts. He
can only do this because he has first differentiated the
separate muscles controlling head movement and has differentiated the results when each muscle is flexed or extended.

Integration of Movements

These separate movements are then integrated as the infant voluntarily executes a pattern of movement to achieve a particular objective. Any particular integration results in a pattern which reflects the intention of the organism. Once all the basic differentiated movements are known, an almost infinite variety of combinations (integrations) are possible.

Generalization of Movement

Large numbers of tasks requiring similar muscle movements may be achieved by generalizing a set of particular patterns (integrations) to them all. For instance, a walking movement generalizes to all other forms of bipedal locomotion; roller skating will generalize to ice-skating and to cross-country skiing; typing and piano playing have some things in common.

THE ANISA CURRICULUM FOR THE DEVELOPMENT

OF PSYCHO-MOTOR COMPETENCE

For the purpose of establishing a curriculum for the development of psycho-motor competence, we have identified a number of basic processes which underlie learning competence in the psycho-motor area. While our focus will be primarily on the psycho-motor area, it should be borne in mind that development in this area is closely associated with perceptual development. For example, hand movements developmentally lead the eyes. Later, a child will utilize his eyes to give him the information he needs to direct his hand. Psycho-motor and perceptual development are given separate treatment in the Anisa process curriculum for the purposes of achieving conceptual clarity.

The Anisa theory of curriculum defines curriculum as two interrelated sets of goals (process goals which are related to the attainment of learning competence and content goals which concern information about the environments verbally and mathematically coded and stored in the memory) and what children and teachers do (how they interact with the environment) to achieve these goals. In the interests of brevity we will emphasize here the definition of the process goals related to the development of psycho-motor competence while the content goals and the precise explanation of what

teachers and children do in terms of activities to achieve
both content and process goals will not be dealt with in any
detail. Furthermore, a number of important issues are
beyond the scope of this article: discussion of muscle
strength; growth spurts in muscular development; sex and
age differences related to strength, growth spurts, and
endurance; fatigue factors; and, the physiology of muscle
contraction.

We define psycho-motor competence as an inner awareness of all of the muscles (which can come under voluntary
control to whatever degree), all of the differentiated movements of body parts they are capable of affecting, and the
ability to execute an infinite variety of combinations
(integrations) of such movements into patterns which express
purposes of the organism. By "body parts" we mean more than
head, limbs, and trunk; included are muscles which control
the size of blood vessels, muscles which move the eyes, the
tongue, the lips, the bladder and anal sphincters, the
muscles producing speech sounds, muscles which comprise the
genital organs, and the diaphragm which controls breathing.
For the sake of completeness, our list of movement patterns
includes those relative to muscles whose differentiations
and integrations come about largely through maturation and
for which little conscious learning is required. However,
although a minimum functioning for many of the muscles
which sustain the vital functions (circulation, respiration,
digestion, elimination, and reproduction) comes about primarily through maturation, the movement of such muscles
can, through practice come under more voluntary control than
is ordinarily achieved and in some cases (i.e., reduction
of blood pressure) the physical health of the organism can
be improved through the extension of voluntary control to a
number of these muscles.

Through his movements, the infant comes to separate or
differentiate all of the muscles (in proximal-distal and
cephalo-caudal directions) and eventually achieves control
over a variety of movement patterns which represent generali-
zable integrations of the differentiated movements. The
proprioceptive organs in muscles, tendons, ligaments, and
joints provide direct information about the status of muscles and their possible movements. The bits of information
coming from the proprioceptors are accumulated as the child
experiences the movement of body parts and muscles. These
bits of information are organized into structures which
constitute the emerging inner awareness of all of the

187

possibilities for muscular movement. Kephart (1971) and Early (1969) call this internally organized structure of motor information the motor base. Kephart emphasizes that if differentiation is incomplete or if differentiation has occurred out of sequence (i.e., integrations are forced before differentiations have been made), the child may develop "splintered" skills in which the movements are angular, rigid, and involve muscular strain. Splintering often occurs when a fine motor skill (such as writing) is required of a child before all of the gross motor skills involving the same muscles required by writing have been developed. In working with slow learners, Kephart became convinced that many learning disorders result from an inadequately structured motor base.

Muscle movements throughout the body are coordinated to perform categories of functions pertinent to different systems. We have therefore organized many of the basic processes underlying psycho-motor competence in terms of these systems. The following muscle systems perform a variety of functions which depend on patterned movements of muscles. These movements reflect the processes which comprise the basic structure of the motor base on which psycho-motor competence depends.

I. Vital Functions-Systems (movement patterns of these muscles are largely determined by reflex action and maturation rather than consciously directed learning.)

    A. Respiratory system.

        All movement patterns of muscles involved in breathing (primarily the diaphragm, muscles involved in the movement of the ribs, throat, and nasal passages.)

    B. Circulatory system.

        Cardiac functioning

        Vasomotor activity (dialation and constriction of blood vessels.)

    C. Digestive system.

        Includes all movement patterns of muscles used in chewing, swallowing, breaking down the food (stomach) assimilating nutrients (intestines) and elimination.

D. Reproductive system.

Movement patterns of muscles of the male and female genitals and muscles in the uterine walls.

II. Skeletal Muscle System

A. Balance and posture. The ability to maintain balance and posture through accommodation (movement) to the forces of gravity while maintaining a position in space.

1. Verticality. Functional awareness of different muscles and their movements and their relationship to the direction of gravity; awareness of what neuro-muscular operations (integrations) are required to stabilize the body with reference to this direction (verticality); this includes the awareness of which muscles are "up" and which ones are "down" and how to move the required muscles to maintain stability.

2. Laterality. Functional awareness that the body has sides: right and left (symmetrical laterality) and dorsal and ventral (asymmetrical laterality).

3. Directionality. Functional awareness of the integration of verticality and laterality and their corresponding movement patterns to maintain the organism in its relationship to the forces of gravity. Different combinations of verticality and laterality are reflected in movement patterns which are recognized as sitting, standing, lying down, bending over, kneeling, etc. Generalization from this internal organization to the external environment involves perceptual and cognitive functions which set the stage for the development of locomotion, or movement of the organism from place to place within the physical environment.

B. Locomotion. The ability to execute a series of muscular movements over time through space while maintaining balance and posture. While balance and posture are being attained, mastery over locomotion

189

emerges as a dominant goal of the organism. Sub-processes of locomotion are:

1.   Sequence. The ability to organize the movement of body parts in an ordered series (culminating in such activities as walking or swimming).

2.   Synchrony. The capacity to control simultan-movements of body parts.

3.   Rhythm. The ability to perform a regular succession of repeated motor actions.

4.   Pace (velocity and acceleration). The ability to establish appropriate timing of locomotor movements appropriate to given intensions of the organism.

Various combinations of the above sub-processes yield different patterns of locomotion: crawling, walking, jumping, hopping, diving, swimming, running, skipping, galloping, skiing, skating. Both balance and posture are prerequisites of locomotion.

C.   Manipulation.

1.   Making contact.

a.   Reaching and grasping

b.   Receipt (catching)

2.   Maintaining contact (holding).

3.   Handling (squeezing/rubbing/piercing/rolling/guiding).

4.   Terminating contact.

a.   Releasing or dropping

b.   Propulsion (throwing)

All of the above are accomplished either when the organism as a whole is stationary or when it is moving (during locomotion) and includes the use of objects as extensions of the body (as in the use of a hammar or other tools). The basic differentiations in skeletal muscle movements may be classified as flexions, extensions, and rotations. Integrations of these among any combination of muscles and/or muscle groups make up the patterned movements that reflect psycho-motor competence.

III. Speech System

A. Movement of muscles in patterns which propel air through vocal chords (primarily the diaphragm).

B. Movement patterns of the muscles of the pharynx and larynx involved in the production of sound (vocal chords) and the alteration of pitch, amplitude, and timbre.

C. Movement patterns of the muscles involved in articulation (facial muscles, throat muscles, muscles of the jaw, tongue, lips and throat).

IV. Perceptual Systems

A variety of muscles are used to support perception through different modalities. Among the most important set of muscles are those concerned with visual perception:

A. Eyelid movements (open, close, squint)

B. Eyeball movements (circular, vertical, horizontal)

C. Lens accommodation (flatten or thicken to provide focus on far or near objects).

The Anisa model is functionally defined by specifications which explain the processes that underlie learning competence and describe the kinds of activities or expeiences children must have in order to develop the processes. Thus, specifications on processes which pertain to the fundamental patterned movements in each of the above systems explicate the process-curriculum in the psycho-motor category of potentialities. When, through learning, these potentialities are actualized, they become the psycho-motor powers of the person--energy expressed in the form of patterned movement.

These powers, of course, are not independent from other functions of the organism; they are inextricably bound up with perceptual, cognitive, affective, and volitional powers as well. For example, the motor base forms the foundation on which other sense impressions are organized. Thus, the structure of the motor base has an effect upon the organization of sensory input and therefore an effect on perception. Concepts are fairly dependent in large part on percepts. The richness of percepts and their availability at any given moment therefore have a bearing upon cognitive competence. Researchers have demonstrated that psycho-motor development is related to the child's ability to express feelings and emotions. The movement of muscles involved in articulate speech as well as a variety of facial expressions and gestures all help to communicate information about our emotional state. Thus, psycho-motor competence has a bearing upon the attainment of affective competence. Since the movement of muscles is purposive on some level, psycho-motor competence heavily implicates volitional development and vice versa.

Finally, the child's feelings about himself are in large part composed of how he feels about his body's appearance, the quality of its movements and capabilities (Buchanan, 1970; Hanson, 1970; Secard & Jouard, 1953). The feeling of comfort that comes from a sense of poise has an influence on one's general confidence for it brings to the organism a sense of general competence. Such a sense of competence gives rise to a sense of self-worth which is important to social maturity and the ability to establish and maintain satisfactory social relations.

Psycho-motor competence is also heavily implicated in achieving technological competence (man as a tool-user), moral competence (because of its role in achieving poise and the ability to communicate effectively), and spiritual competence (because of the relationship between confidence and security--which have roots in psycho-motor competency--and the ability to approach unknowns on faith). Finally, the learning of symbol systems (e.g., reading and writing or sign language) depends upon the coordinate patterns of various muscle movements.

But perhaps most important of all is the fact that the general development of the organism rests upon the interaction with the environment and the primary modality of interacting with the environment depends upon the movement of muscles. Thus, the release of all human potentialities at an optimum rate rests heavily upon the individual's psycho-motor powers, hence the primary accord given to their development in the Anisa model.

REFERENCES

Bayley, N. "The development of motor abilities during the first three years." Monog. Soc. Res. Child Development, 1935, I, 1-26.

Buchanan, E. The relationship of affective behavior to movement patterns, body image, and visual perception. Doctoral dissertation, University of California, Los Angeles, 1970.

Cratty, B. J. Perceptual and motor development in infants and children. New York: Macmillan & Co., 1970.

Early. G. H. Perceptual training in the curriculum. Columbus, Ohio: Charles E. Merrill Publishing Co., 1969.

Gardner, E. Fundamentals of neurology. Philadelphia: W. B. Saunders & Co., 1958.

Gesell, A. Studies in child development. New York: Harper Brothers, 1948.

Hanson, D. S. The effect of a concentrated program in movement behavior on the affective behavior of four year old children at University Elementary School. Doctoral dissertation, University of California, 1970.

Kephart, N. C. The slow learner in the classroom. (2nd Ed.) Columbus, Ohio: Charles E. Merrill Publishing Co., 1969.

McGraw, M. B. The neuromuscular maturation of the human infant. New York: Hafner Pub. Co., Inc., 1943.

Shirley, M. M. "The first two years: A study of twenty-five babies." Vol. I. Postural and locomotor development. Minneapolis: University of Minnesota Press, 1931.

Secard, P., & Jourard, S. "The appraisal of body-cathexis: Body cathexis and the self." J. Consult. Psychol., 1953, 17, 343-7.

Whitehead, A. N. Aims of education. New York: Macmillan Co., 1967.

A CRITIQUE OF PIAGET'S THEORY OF THE ONTOGENESIS OF MOTOR BEHAVIOR

DAVID P. AUSUBEL

A. INTRODUCTION

In recent years, Piaget's formulations regarding the ontogenesis of motor behavior during the first 18 months of life have won a wide measure of acceptance from child psychologists everywhere—even from American authors [e.g., Hunt (6) and Flavell (3)] who have hitherto tended to be highly critical of both his theories and his methodology. One of Piaget's basic assumptions about early motor development is that there is functional comparability and developmental continuity between reflex and nonreflex behavioral sequences. For example, he derives more advanced forms of cortically controlled prehension (e.g., primary circular reactions, hand-mouth coordinations, visual-manual coordinations) from the primitive, subcortically regulated grasping reflex via such mechanisms as "generalizing assimilation," "differential assimilation," and "reciprocal assimilation" to the "grasping schema" (9, pp. 89-116). The theoretical difficulty here arises from the paradoxical fact that Piaget of all persons, who ordinarily overelaborates stage differences far beyond his data, appears to ignore the fundamental distinction between reflex and nonreflex activity. As a result, his description and explanation of early motor development obscure basic differences in rate, patterning, and regulation characteristic of these two forms of behavior, as well as the salient generalization that motor development, as it is generally understood, is an outgrowth of nonreflex rather than of reflex activity [see Ausubel (1, p. 206)]. This theoretical difficulty, of course, applies less to such developmental sequences as sucking and visual pursuit movements that are nonreflex in nature from the very beginning than to sequences that are reflex in nature from the very beginning.

Widespread uncritical acceptance in the United States of Piaget's views concerning the ontogenesis of motor behavior is somewhat surprising considering (a) the well-established distinction between reflex and nonreflex (instrumental, voluntary) behavior that has traditionally prevailed both among Amer-

JOURNAL OF GENETIC PSYCHOLOGY, 1966, Vol. 109, pp. 119-122.

ican psychologists generally and among American students of early motor development (2, 4, 7, 8, 10), and (*b*) the widely accepted Skinnerian distinction between respondent and operant behavior.

B. Neonatal Differences

From the very beginning of neonatal life, reflex and nonreflex behavior are distinguishably different. The stimulus-response connections of reflex behavior are more strongly predetermined by genic factors and are more specific and invariable than those of nonreflex behavior. Reflex acts are also elicited by more particular and specifiable stimuli, and are more adaptive and relevant in relation to the stimuli that evoke them than are nonreflex acts; in any case, their adaptiveness is more innately determined than a product of learning. On the other hand, even relatively localized and segmental nonreflex responses (e.g., sucking) can be triggered off by completely irrelevant stimuli; and, conversely, a single stimulus may evoke several irrelevant as well as relevant nonreflex responses. Whereas individuation of reflex activity virtually reaches completion at birth, individuation of nonreflex activity is at best minimal. Most of the integrated behavior displayed by the neonate consists of coordinated reflexes, such as subcortically controlled creeping and swimming movements and the Moro reflex. Thus the general picture of neonatal behavioral organization is epitomized by the striking contrast between the highly developed segmental and coordinated reflexes and the relatively diffuse, amorphous nonreflex responses that have yet to be individuated and coordinated.

Of particular importance is the distinction between spinal and subcortical regulation of reflex activity, on the one hand, and cortical regulation of nonreflex activity, on the other. Neonatal nonreflex behavior is amorphous in character largely because the degree of cortical control and inhibition that is necessary both for precise and directed specific movements on a nonreflex level, as well as for integration of such movements into increasingly complex patterns, has yet to be attained in the postneonatal period. Cortical inhibition in the first six to 12 months of life is even extended to some *reflexes,* especially to those that are intersegmental in nature (e.g., mass reflex, Moro reflex), and that are suggestive of prehensile (grasp reflex) and locomotor (stepping, swimming, and creeping movements) functions. These latter reflexes are eventually replaced by more segmental or restricted reflexes (e.g., plantar, startle) and by voluntary, cortically controlled prehensile and locomotor responses (8). But except for chronological antecedence and superficial resemblance in the kind of behavior involved, the subcortical, reflex stage of these activities bears little relationship to the cortical, voluntary stage that follows.

The latter is not a functional or developmental outgrowth of the former, but merely a later-occurring phenotypically similar activity dependent upon intervening neural maturation (1, p. 211).

Thus, for example, during the first four to six months of postnatal life, the grasp reflex is gradually replaced by volitional grasping that is both less invariable and characterized by conspicuous involvement of the thumb (5). It is legitimate to interpret this developmental trend as an indication both of increased cortical control and of inhibition of a subcortically regulated reflex, especially since the grasp reflex may be reactivated after injury to the premotor area of the cortex.

C. Subsequent Development

Once maximal specificity is attained shortly after birth, reflex behavior undergoes relatively little change. Except for the few reflexes that are suppressed by cortical inhibition, the neonate's vast repertoire of reflex behavior remains intact throughout the life-span. From time to time, of course, depending upon particular idiosyncratic experience, conditioning may occur. In contrast, individuation of nonreflex behavior, far from being substantially complete during the neonatal period, is a continuing aspect of motor development, both in the early "phylogenetic" phase dominated by neural maturation and in the later "ontogenetic" stages dominated by practice (1, p. 209). Hence most of the behavioral change subsumed under motor development occurs in the area of nonreflex activity. With increasing age, nonreflex responses become increasingly localized, economical in extent of involvement, and relevant in relation to their eliciting stimuli—but never as specific or invariable as true reflexes.

Postneonatal modifications of reflex and nonreflex behavior also follow widely divergent paths. Modifications of reflex activity (classical conditioning) tend to be relatively unadaptive, rigid, and irrelevant in relation to new stimulus content, depending as they do solely on arbitrary contiguity. Modifications of nonreflex activity, on the other hand, are more relevant, adaptive, and flexible products of instrumental learning in which either reinforcement of the successful variant or cognitive appreciation of means-ends relationships plays significant roles. Neonatal nonreflex behavior, furthermore, is the developmental precursor of intentional or voluntary behavior, whereas reflex behavior never acquires intentionality. The latter is stimulus-bound in the sense that it can be initiated only by stimulation, never voluntarily, and is not ordinarily subject to voluntary inhibition.

Finally, Piaget's explanation of motor development in terms of modification

196

(generalizing, differential, and reciprocal assimilation) of original reflex schemata has a strongly nominalistic flavor. His explanations generate an illusion of accounting for the nature and causes of developmental sequences, whereas actually they mostly rephrase simple descriptive analyses into more abstract and highly idiosyncratic language. "Reciprocal assimilation of prehensile and visual schemata," for example, tells us little about the actual development of eye-hand coordination—either about the developmental mechanisms involved or the principal determining variables.

REFERENCES

1. AUSUBEL, D. P. Theory and Problems of Child Development. New York: Grune & Stratton, 1958.
2. DENNIS, W. A description and classification of the responses of the newborn infant. *Psychol. Bull.*, 1934, **31**, 5-22.
3. FLAVELL, J. H. The Developmental Psychology of Jean Piaget. Princeton, N. J.: Van Nostrand, 1963.
4. GESELL, A. The ontogenesis of infant behavior. In L. Carmichael (Ed.), *Manual of Child Psychology* (2nd ed.). New York: Wiley, 1954. Pp. 335-373.
5. HALVERSON, H. M. Studies of the grasping responses of early infancy: I, II, and III. *J. Genet. Psychol.*, 1937, **51**, 371-449.
6. HUNT, J. McV. Intelligence and Experience. New York: Ronald Press, 1961.
7. IRWIN, O. C. The amount and nature of activities of newborn infants under constant external stimulating conditions during the first ten days of life. *Genet. Psychol. Monog.*, 1930, **8**, 1-92.
8. McGRAW, M. B. The Neuromuscular Maturation of the Human Infant. New York: Columbia Univ. Press, 1943.
9. PIAGET, J. The Origins of Intelligence in Children. New York: Internat. Univ. Press, 1952.
10. PRATT, K. C. The neonate. In L. Carmichael (Ed.), *Manual of Child Psychology* (2nd ed.). New York: Wiley, 1954. Pp. 215-291.

APPENDIX
A Summary Statement on the Anisa* Model

The Anisa model represents a comprehensive educational system functionally defined by specifications which insure its replicability, evaluation, and refinement. The specifications set forth educational objectives pertaining to the actualization of human potential and explanations of how to achieve them. These objectives and explanations are derived from a coherent body of theory which has been deductively generated from a philosophical base and inductively validated to whatever extent possible by findings from empirical research.

The philosophy underlying the model is organismic in nature; it defines man as a spiritual as well as a material being; explains his reality in terms of the process of his becoming (actualization of potentiality), accounts for his qualities of transcendence and immanence, and sets forth fundamental ontological principles which explicate man's relationship to the universe.

The body of theory derived from the philosophy includes:

A Theory of Development which defines development as the translation of potentiality into actuality and equates that translation with creativity; establishes two broad categories of potentialities—biological and psychological; identifies proper nutrition as the essential element in the development of biological potentialities and learning as the key factor in the release of psychological potentialities; establishes five categories of psychological potentialities—psycho-motor, perceptual, cognitive, affective, and volitional; establishes interaction with the environment as the means by which development is sustained; fixes three basic categories of environment (physical, human and the unknown) and establishes the Self as the micro-cosmic reflection of the three environments and the most constant aspect of the environment it experiences; and, categorizes interactions in terms of their power to facilitate development and safeguard survival.

A Theory of Curriculum which fixes the overarching goal of education as the actualization of human potentialities and their structuring into identities around ideals which guarantee survival and perpetually improve its quality; establishes two categories of goals or objectives of the

199

formal educational system—content goals and process goals; specifies the substance of the former as the information culture has accumulated organized in terms of the classification of environments, including the symbol systems used to convey that information, and the substance of the latter as formation of internal structures on which learning competence depends (i.e., content goals may specify what to think about, while process goals concentrate on how to think); accounts for the emergence of personal identity (character formation) in terms of value formation and defines values as the relatively enduring structurings of potentialities (process) as they are actualized and integrated with information (content) assimilated about the various environments; and, specifies three value sub-systems (material, social, and religious/aesthetic) on which three higher order competencies rest (technological, moral and spiritual/philosophical) and which combine to form the total values system that constitutes the personality—the Self.

A Theory of Pedagogy which defines teaching as arranging environments and guiding the child's interaction with them for the purpose of achieving the goals specified by the curriculum theory; outlines the diagnostic, prescriptive, speculative, experimental, and improvisational aspects of arranging environments and guiding interaction so that instruction is individualized and learning particularized thereby guaranteeing equality of educational opportunity.

A Theory of Administration which identifies two basic functions of administration which must remain in dynamic equilibrium—leadership and management—and defines them in terms of service consistent with purpose as specified by the philosophy; provides the rationale for differentiating the staff, maintaining morale, establishing institutional priorities, assessing needs, identifying resources, determining feasibility, and allocating resources to achieve objectives as efficiently as possible; provides the means for institutional self-renewal; and, accounts for the necessity and nature of community and home involvement.

A Theory of Evaluation which designates comparative analysis of children's interactions with particular environments and their developmental consequences as the focal point of inquiry; seeks to relate means to ends, distinguishing efficient from final causes; and allies the purpose of evaluation with the heuristic, explanatory, and predictive functions of research and science.

Because the model rests on the universal processes of growth and development, it has cross-cultural applicability and addresses directly the problem of how to achieve equal educational opportunity.

---

* Anisa is both a word and an acronym. As a word, it has Greek and Latin roots which refer to a flowering tree whose fragrance has made it attractive as a symbol. It has been adopted to represent "the tree of life"—an ancient symbol connoting shelter, beauty and grace, and the perpetual growth and fruition of organic life. The tree of life is reflected in the Anisa logogram. As an acronym, Anisa stands for American National Institutes for Social Advancement, an incorporated not-for-profit organization under whose auspices the efforts to formulate the model were undertaken.

Dr. Linda M. Blane is Assistant Professor, Center for the Study of Human Potential, School of Education at the University of Massachusetts. In addition to her teaching and research responsibilities as a member of the graduate faculty, she is a member of the staff working on the development of the ANISA Model.